Contents

Welcome to the *Reboot* series—a comprehensive collection of books designed to explore and demystify the underlying emotional and psychological factors behind some of the most common health challenges we face today. Each book in this series delves deeply into a specific condition, such as prostate health, breast cancer, Fibromyalgia or digestive issues, and may more, offering an integrative approach that combines the latest scientific research with the profound insights of German New Medicine and holistic health practices. Whether you're seeking to prevent illness, support a loved one, or embark on your own healing journey, this series aims to empower you with the knowledge and tools needed to reclaim your health and well-being from within.

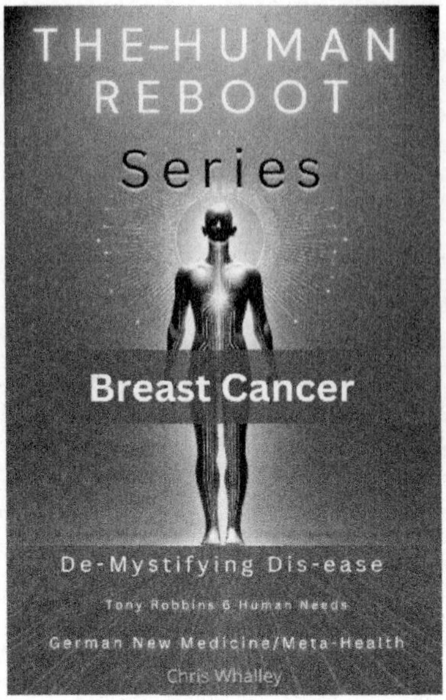
THE-HUMAN
REBOOT
Series
Breast Cancer
De-Mystifying Dis-ease
Tony Robbins 6 Human Needs
German New Medicine/Meta-Health
Chris Whalley

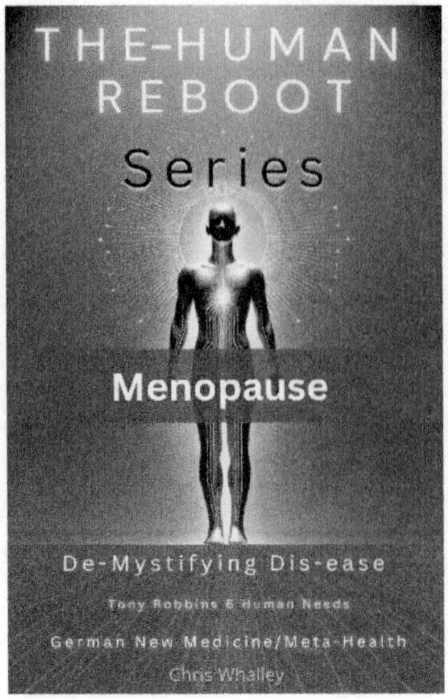
THE-HUMAN
REBOOT
Series
Menopause
De-Mystifying Dis-ease
Tony Robbins 6 Human Needs
German New Medicine/Meta-Health
Chris Whalley

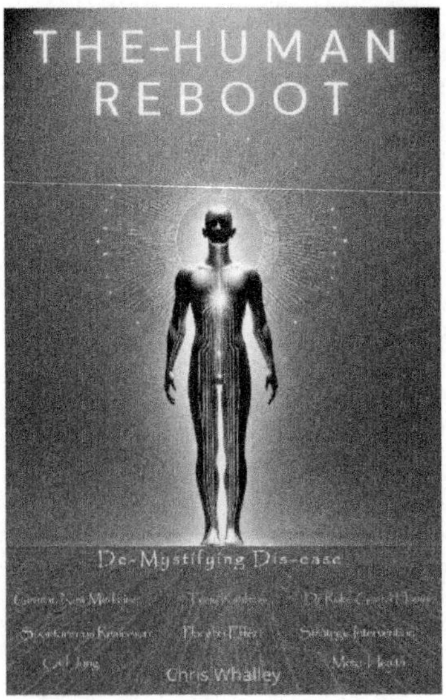
THE-HUMAN
REBOOT
De-Mystifying Dis-ease
Chris Whalley

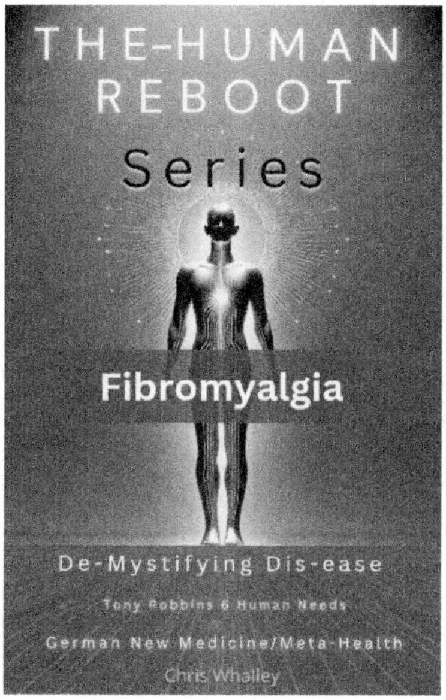
THE-HUMAN
REBOOT
Series
Fibromyalgia
De-Mystifying Dis-ease
Tony Robbins 6 Human Needs
German New Medicine/Meta-Health
Chris Whalley

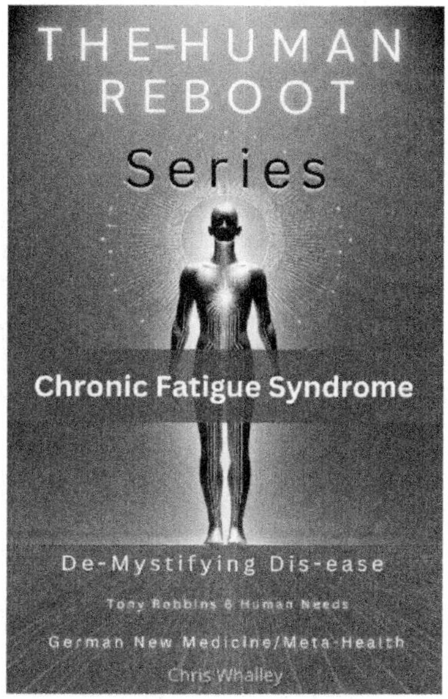
THE-HUMAN
REBOOT
Series
Chronic Fatigue Syndrome
De-Mystifying Dis-ease
Tony Robbins 6 Human Needs
German New Medicine/Meta-Health
Chris Whalley

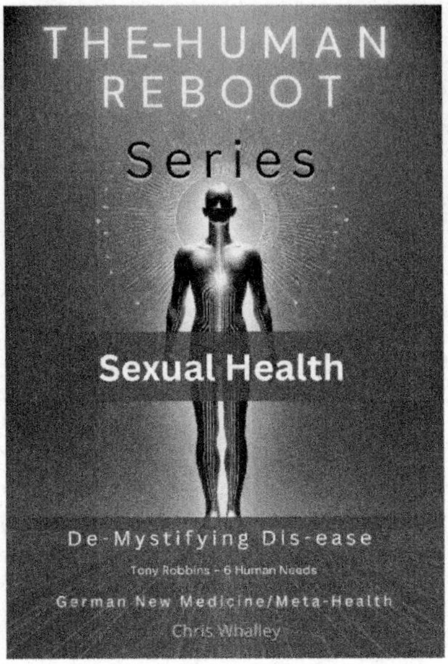
THE-HUMAN REBOOT
Series
Sexual Health
De-Mystifying Dis-ease
Tony Robbins - 6 Human Needs
German New Medicine/Meta-Health
Chris Whalley

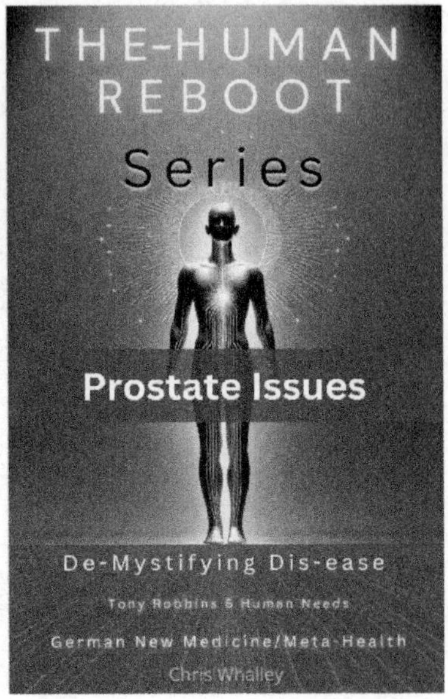
THE-HUMAN REBOOT
Series
Prostate Issues
De-Mystifying Dis-ease
Tony Robbins 6 Human Needs
German New Medicine/Meta-Health
Chris Whalley

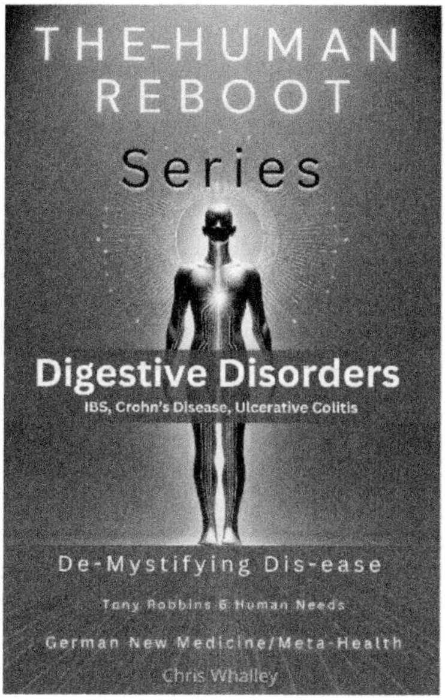
THE-HUMAN
REBOOT
Series
Digestive Disorders
IBS, Crohn's Disease, Ulcerative Colitis
De-Mystifying Dis-ease
Tony Robbins & Human Needs
German New Medicine/Meta-Health
Chris Whalley

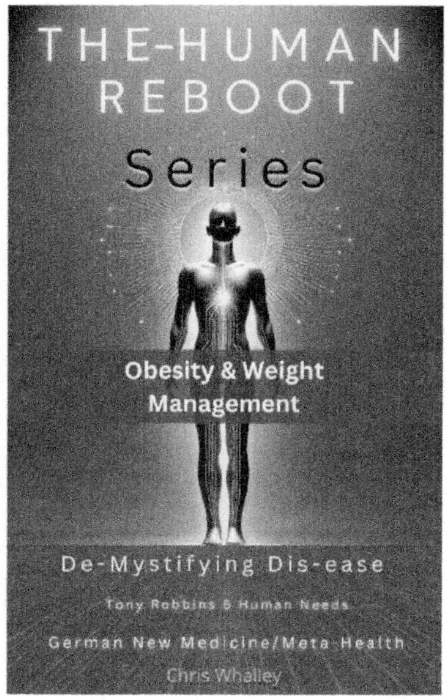
THE-HUMAN
REBOOT
Series
Obesity & Weight
Management
De-Mystifying Dis-ease
Tony Robbins & Human Needs
German New Medicine/Meta-Health
Chris Whalley

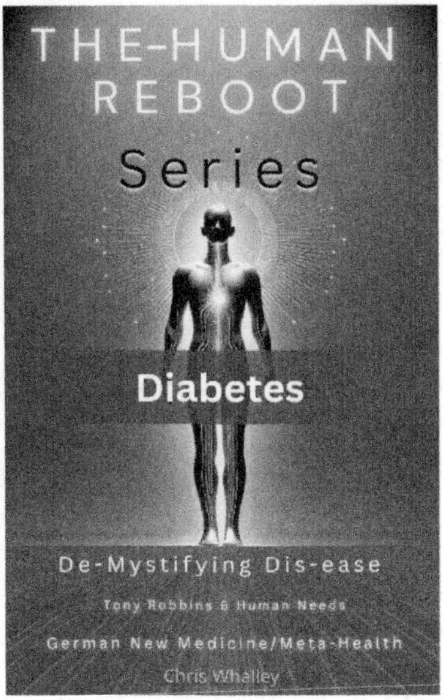
THE-HUMAN
REBOOT
Series
Diabetes
De-Mystifying Dis-ease
Tony Robbins 6 Human Needs
German New Medicine/Meta-Health
Chris Whalley
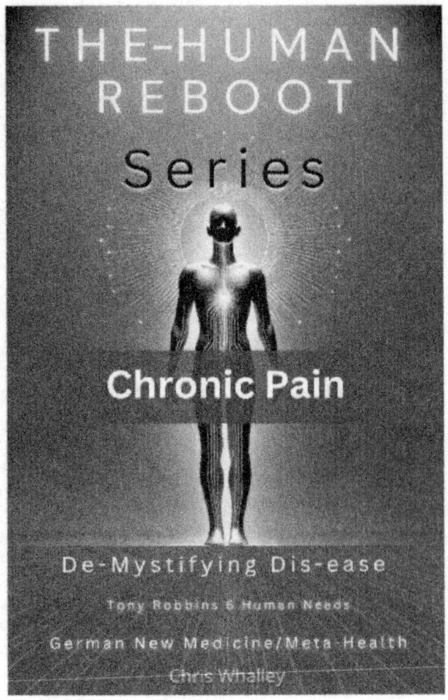
THE-HUMAN
REBOOT
Series
Chronic Pain
De-Mystifying Dis-ease
Tony Robbins 6 Human Needs
German New Medicine/Meta-Health
Chris Whalley

Disclaimer:

The information presented in this book is intended for educational and informational purposes only. It is not intended as a substitute for professional medical advice, diagnosis, or treatment. Always seek the advice of your physician or other qualified health provider with any questions you may have regarding a medical condition. Never disregard professional medical advice or delay seeking it because of something you have read in this book.

The author and publisher of this book are not responsible for any health issues that may arise from the application of information contained herein. The content is based on the author's research, opinions, and personal experiences and is not intended to diagnose, treat, or prevent any disease.

All efforts have been made to ensure the accuracy of the information provided, but the author and publisher assume no responsibility for errors, omissions, or contradictory information. The reader is encouraged to verify any information presented in this book and to consult a healthcare professional before making any changes to their health regimen.

Welcome!

The book you're holding is an important step in your journey, offering powerful insights to guide your growth and understanding. But what if I told you there's a way to unlock even more?

Human Reboot is the cornerstone of the *Reboot* series—the master guide that connects all the dots. It delves deeper into the principles, frameworks, and life-changing insights that underpin everything you'll find in this book and more.

Readers have described *Human Reboot* as 'life-changing,' revealing truths that empower them to not only understand their challenges but overcome them with confidence and clarity.

Why settle for just part of the picture? Dive into the full story and discover how *Human Reboot* can transform your health, mindset, and life.

Start your journey now—grab your copy of *Human Reboot* at https://mybook.to/StkDuTx

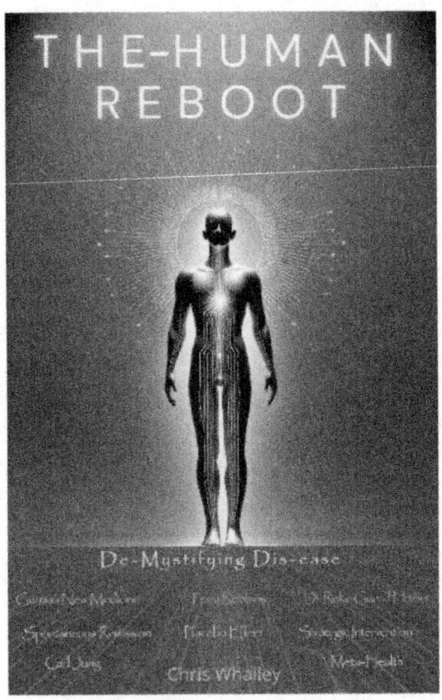

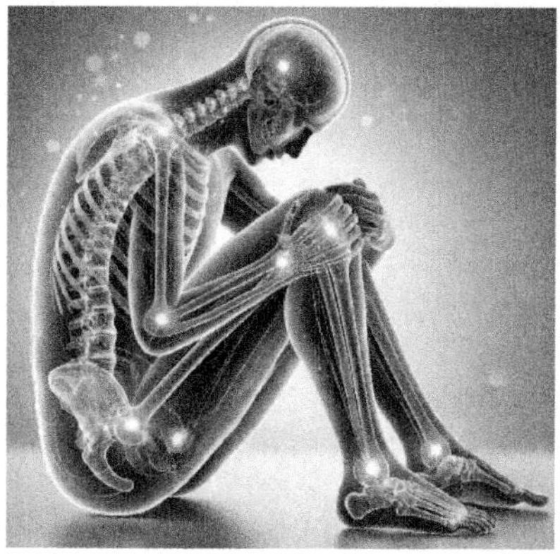

Introduction: A New Understanding of Health and Healing

Imagine for a moment that your body is not broken. Imagine that everything it does—even the pain, the fatigue, and the seemingly endless symptoms—is part of a meaningful process, one designed to help you survive. This book invites you to consider a completely new perspective on health and disease, especially when it comes to fibromyalgia.

To illustrate this approach, picture your body as a house. Over time, cracks may appear in the walls, or the foundation might weaken due to stressors like weather or wear and tear. When emotional stress is unresolved, it's as though scaffolding surrounds the house, protecting and reinforcing the structure. However, if the underlying cause—the emotional conflict—is not addressed, that scaffolding remains indefinitely, creating further imbalance. This book will guide you in understanding fibromyalgia's symptoms, not as malfunctions, but as part of your body's natural attempt to heal and strengthen itself.

Let's begin with a story that reshaped how we understand illness and illustrates the profound connection between emotional stress and physical symptoms.

The Story of Dr. Ryke Geerd Hamer

In 1978, Dr. Ryke Geerd Hamer, a successful physician, experienced a life-altering emotional shock. His teenage son, Dirk, was tragically injured in an accident and later died from his injuries. The loss was devastating. Just months later, Dr. Hamer was diagnosed with testicular cancer.

As both a doctor and a grieving father, he began to wonder if the emotional trauma of losing his son had triggered his illness. Determined to find answers, he conducted extensive research, uncovering a groundbreaking understanding of disease that would later become known as **German New Medicine (GNM).**

Why Testicular Cancer?

Dr. Hamer's diagnosis of testicular cancer was not random. According to GNM, diseases are not malfunctions but biologically meaningful responses to intense emotional conflicts. In his case, the death of his son represented a **biological conflict of loss**, tied to reproduction and the survival of his lineage.

The testicles play a key role in reproduction, ensuring the continuation of one's bloodline. When Dr. Hamer experienced the devastating loss of his son, his subconscious registered this as a profound threat to his family's future. Biologically, his body activated a **special biological program** to adapt to this loss. This program involved cell proliferation in the testicular tissue—an effort to increase reproductive capacity and secure the continuation of his lineage.

This process wasn't a malfunction; it was a survival mechanism deeply rooted in evolution. However, because the emotional conflict remained unresolved, his body stayed in a state of **hanging healing**, unable to complete the biological program. This discovery formed the foundation of GNM, which explains how emotional conflicts impact the **psyche**, the **brain**, and specific **tissues or organs**, leading to symptoms.

A New Perspective on Symptoms

GNM reframes our understanding of symptoms as purposeful, biologically meaningful processes. For example, just as Dr. Hamer's testicular cancer was his body's adaptive response to the loss of his son, fibromyalgia symptoms like chronic pain and fatigue can be seen as the body's attempt to manage prolonged emotional stress—particularly **self-devaluation conflicts.**

Self-devaluation often involves feelings of inadequacy, worthlessness, or failure. In fibromyalgia, these emotional conflicts manifest physically, as the body breaks down and rebuilds tissues in an effort to adapt and strengthen.

However, if the conflicts remain unresolved, the body becomes trapped in a cycle of **hanging healing**, where symptoms persist as part of the ongoing biological program.

Shadows and Archetypes: Understanding the Emotional Component

While emotional conflicts trigger biological responses, unresolved psychological patterns often keep the cycle going. In this book, we'll explore these patterns through the lens of **shadow selves** and **archetypes**—hidden parts of ourselves that influence our behaviors and relationships.

There are four primary shadows we may embody:

- **Blamer:** Deflects responsibility onto others, avoiding feelings of inadequacy.
- **Placator:** Sacrifices their own needs to gain approval or avoid conflict.
- **Computer:** Detaches from emotions, relying solely on logic to avoid vulnerability.
- **Distractor:** Avoids dealing with deeper issues by creating chaos or using humour as a shield.

Each shadow has an empowered counterpart, or archetype:

- The **Blamer** can evolve into the **Warrior**, who takes responsibility and acts with courage and integrity.
- The **Placator** can become the **Lover**, who nurtures themselves and others without sacrificing their identity.
- The **Computer** can transform into the **Guru**, who balances intellect with emotional wisdom.
- The **Distractor** can become the **Jester**, who uses humour constructively while staying emotionally present.

Throughout this book, you'll learn how these shadows and archetypes relate to your emotional and physical health. By understanding and transforming these patterns, you can begin to address the root causes of your symptoms.

The Drama Triangle and Fibromyalgia

Another key concept we'll explore is the **Drama Triangle**, a model describing unhealthy relationship dynamics. In these dynamics, individuals often adopt one of three roles:

- **Victim:** Feels powerless and blames others or external circumstances.
- **Rescuer:** Tries to fix others' problems, often at their own expense.
- **Persecutor:** Criticizes or blames others to maintain control.

These roles can perpetuate emotional stress, keeping the body in a state of hanging healing. Recognizing your role within the Drama Triangle is an essential step toward breaking free from these patterns and fostering healthier relationships with yourself and others.

Moving Forward: A New Way of Seeing Disease

German New Medicine teaches us that disease is not a malfunction but a biologically intelligent process. Your symptoms are not random; they are your body's attempt to cope with unresolved emotional conflicts. For example, if you've felt devalued or unsupported for years, your body may respond with pain and fatigue as part of its effort to protect and heal you.

By identifying and resolving these underlying conflicts, you can break free from the cycle of chronic symptoms. It's like finally removing the scaffolding from a house once the repairs are complete. This book is not just about managing fibromyalgia—it's about uncovering the emotional roots of your symptoms and working with your body to restore balance and vitality.

Quick Reference Guide to German New Medicine (GNM) Terms

To help you navigate the concepts in this book, here's a brief guide to key GNM terms:

- **Biological Conflict:** A sudden, unexpected emotional shock that impacts the psyche, brain, and body.
- **DHS (Dirk Hamer Syndrome):** The initial shock that triggers a biological conflict, named after Dr. Hamer's son.

- **Healing Phase:** The stage following conflict resolution, where the body repairs tissues, often causing temporary symptoms like pain and fatigue.
- **Hanging Healing:** When unresolved or recurring conflicts keep the body in a prolonged cycle of stress and healing.

An Invitation to Healing

This book invites you to see your health in a new light. Fibromyalgia is not a random malfunction; it's a biologically meaningful response to unresolved emotional stress. Through understanding GNM, shadow selves, and the Drama Triangle, you'll gain the tools to address the root causes of your symptoms and unlock your body's natural potential for healing.

You'll discover that your body is not broken, and neither are you. By working with your body—rather than against it—you can find balance, resilience, and true healing.

Sam's Story: Overwhelm, Conflict, and Fibromyalgia

Sam Dobson's journey with fibromyalgia began long before her diagnosis. A dedicated mother and professional, Sam's life was a whirlwind of work, home duties, and personal aspirations. Like many, she felt the pressure to succeed—both at work and as a mother—leading her into a cycle of stress and emotional strain.

Working at a high-stress corporate job, Sam was constantly striving to prove herself, balancing the demands of her career with the responsibilities of home life. She suppressed her own needs, believing that working harder and pleasing others would eventually bring fulfillment. Over time, the emotional toll became too great, and her body began signalling distress in the form of aches, fatigue, and chronic pain.

The Build-Up of Emotional Conflict

By the end of 2010, the signs of emotional and physical exhaustion were undeniable. Sam's intense drive to succeed in her career, alongside her role as a mother, had left her with little time to care for her own well-being. She described juggling so many roles that her own health became less of a priority, which made her feel trapped in an endless cycle of overwork. Her body was giving her warning signs—aches, fatigue, and sensitivity—but she didn't understand them at the time.

In January 2011, everything came to a halt. One morning, Sam woke up and couldn't get out of bed. Her body had completely shut down. She described being in so much pain that she couldn't move, and her senses became overwhelmed by even the smallest stimuli—light, noise, and movement. This physical shutdown was a culmination of years of emotional stress, self-devaluation, and feeling unsupported at work and in life.

A New Understanding of Disease through German New Medicine (GNM)

From a **German New Medicine (GNM)** perspective, Sam's fibromyalgia wasn't a random malfunction but a response to the **self-devaluation conflict** she had been experiencing. GNM explains that when we devalue ourselves—constantly thinking we are not good enough, strong enough, or worthy enough—our bodies go through a biological process of tissue breakdown and repair.

Sam's body was breaking down muscle and tissue to rebuild it, in an attempt to make her stronger. However, the emotional conflict remained unresolved, so her body stayed stuck in a cycle of breakdown and attempted healing. This back-and-forth process, known in GNM as **hanging healing**, happens when emotional conflicts are not fully resolved, keeping the body from completing its healing process.

Think of the body as a house under renovation. When a house becomes unstable, scaffolding is put up to support it while repairs are being made. In Sam's case, her body began breaking down tissues to rebuild them stronger, just like the scaffolding. However, because the underlying emotional conflicts weren't fully addressed, the scaffolding never came down, leaving her body in a constant state of attempted healing.

Self-Devaluation and the Placator Shadow

Sam's story also reflects the **Placator shadow**—a part of her that constantly sacrificed her own needs to avoid conflict and gain approval from others. She always put others first, thinking that this would lead to success and happiness. However, this self-sacrifice caused her to suppress her emotions and devalue her own worth, leading to physical symptoms.

Her pattern of overwork, driven by a need to please others and achieve, left her emotionally drained. The Placator shadow kept her in a cycle of seeking external validation, preventing her from recognizing her own value. This self-devaluation was the root cause of her fibromyalgia, as her body responded to her emotional pain by breaking down and rebuilding tissue in an attempt to protect her.

Hanging Healing and Cycles of Stress

After her physical collapse, Sam spent months searching for answers, undergoing various tests, and waiting for diagnoses. The healthcare system, while well-intentioned, couldn't find a clear solution for her symptoms. It wasn't until she began addressing the underlying emotional conflicts—through coaching and self-reflection—that she started to understand the connection between her emotional state and her physical health.

Sam's body was stuck in a state of **hanging healing**, a concept from GNM that describes how the body cannot fully heal while emotional conflicts remain unresolved. The pain, stiffness, and fatigue were not random, but part of her body's ongoing attempt to repair the tissue damage caused by her self-devaluation. Each time she was triggered by stress or emotional strain, her body would revert to the conflict-active phase, preventing full recovery.

Moving from Placator to Lover

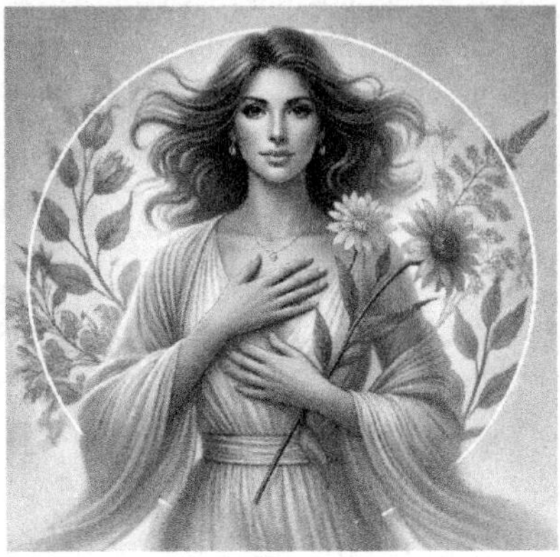

Through our coaching sessions, Sam began to recognize that her value wasn't dependent on others' approval. She learned to step into the empowered version of the **Placator**—the **Lover** archetype.

The **Lover** represents deep compassion, emotional connection, and nurturing, but unlike the Placator, the Lover does not sacrifice themselves in the process. The Lover knows that true love and connection come from a place of balance—the integration of both masculine and feminine energies. The masculine energy of the Lover is seen in setting boundaries and maintaining personal integrity, while the feminine energy shines through in their ability to offer love and empathy, not only to others but also to themselves.

One day, during one of our sessions, Sam had a breakthrough.

"Sam, imagine yourself truly embodying the Lover. What would that look like?" I asked.

She paused, her expression softening, "It would feel like freedom. I'd be able to say no without feeling guilty. I'd finally have space for myself."

From that moment on, Sam began to embrace the Lover archetype—nurturing herself as much as she nurtured others. She realized that self-love and care were vital not just for her well-being but for the health of her relationships as well.

Steps to Empowerment:

- **Set Boundaries with Love**: Begin by identifying areas where you tend to over-sacrifice. How can you start setting healthy boundaries in a way that respects both your needs and the needs of others?
- **Practice Self-Love**: The Lover's strength comes from a deep sense of self-worth. How can you incorporate practices of self-care and self-love into your daily routine?
- **Nurture Without Self-Sacrifice**: Learn to give and receive love in a balanced way. The empowered Lover nurtures others but never at the expense of their own emotional and physical well-being.

Visualize Your Transformation:

Picture yourself as the empowered **Lover**—someone who nurtures and cares deeply, but who also knows their own value. Visualize creating loving, healthy relationships where both you and the people around you feel supported. This is the path of the Lover—where love for self and others leads to true empowerment.

Rachel's Story: Conflict, Resentment, and Chronic Pain

Rachel had always been known for her strong personality and her need to control situations. Whether at work or in her personal life, she often took charge, but her leadership came with a high price—resentment and blame. If things went wrong, she was quick to point fingers, believing that others were the source of her frustration. This constant externalization of conflict masked her own deep-seated feelings of inadequacy, which she had suppressed for years.

Rachel's story illustrates the **Blamer** shadow—a defence mechanism that projects responsibility onto others to avoid facing internal insecurities. Over time, her unresolved emotions began manifesting physically, and her body started to break down, leaving her with chronic pain, fatigue, and a diagnosis of fibromyalgia.

The Conflict Shock (DHS)

The turning point for Rachel came when she lost a major contract at work due to a mistake by one of her team members. The feelings of betrayal and failure were overwhelming, triggering a **self-devaluation conflict** tied to her perceived lack of control. German New Medicine explains that when we feel inadequate or unable to manage a situation, our bodies react by breaking down tissue in an attempt to rebuild it stronger. In Rachel's case, the conflict caused her musculoskeletal system to weaken, leading to chronic pain in her joints and muscles.

Her body's response to this emotional shock wasn't random; it was a biological adaptation designed to help her become stronger. However, because the underlying conflict of self-devaluation wasn't resolved, her body remained in a state of **hanging healing**—a cycle of pain and attempted recovery.

Hanging Healing and Cycles of Stress

Following this major career setback, Rachel's body entered a phase of ongoing stress, unable to fully heal due to recurring emotional triggers. Each time she encountered a new challenge or felt criticized, her body would react with pain and fatigue. She cycled between moments of recovery and relapse, never fully understanding why her symptoms persisted.

From the perspective of **German New Medicine**, Rachel's musculoskeletal issues were not a malfunction but part of her body's attempt to cope with the deep feelings of self-blame and inadequacy. The **Blamer** shadow had her constantly deflecting responsibility, but her body was breaking down and rebuilding tissue to prepare her to face the emotional conflict she was avoiding.

Moving from Blamer to Warrior

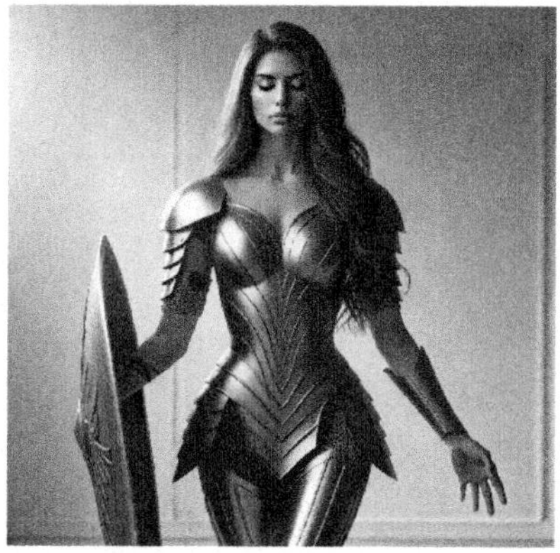

Rachel's journey didn't end with the Blamer shadow defining her life. Through coaching and introspection, she began to recognize that blaming others wasn't solving her problems—it was deepening her physical and emotional struggles. With this realization, Rachel started transitioning into the **Warrior** archetype—the empowered version of the Blamer.

The **Warrior** is someone who takes responsibility for their own actions, thoughts, and feelings. Rather than projecting conflict outward, the Warrior confronts challenges head-on, with courage and integrity. The Warrior's strength doesn't just come from fighting external battles; it also comes from self-awareness, recognizing vulnerabilities, and facing internal struggles with resilience.

I remember one coaching session with Rachel where her shift from Blamer to Warrior became clear.

"Rachel, what would happen if, instead of blaming others, you embraced your own power to change the situation?" I asked.

She paused and replied, "It would mean I'm no longer a victim. I can take control of my own life."

From that point forward, Rachel began embracing the Warrior archetype—taking ownership of her actions and shifting her perspective. She stopped projecting her frustrations onto others and instead focused on building her own emotional strength. This shift wasn't just emotional; her physical symptoms began to improve as well.

Steps to Empowerment:

- **Take Responsibility**: Reflect on areas in your life where you tend to blame others for outcomes. Ask yourself, "What part of this do I have control over, and how can I take responsibility for my role?"
- **Face Challenges with Courage**: The Warrior doesn't shy away from conflict but confronts it directly. How can you begin facing your personal and professional challenges with strength and integrity?
- **Balance Strength and Vulnerability**: True power comes from within. The Warrior embraces both strength and vulnerability, using their energy to find solutions while remaining open to growth and healing.

Visualize Your Transformation:

Imagine yourself as the empowered **Warrior**—someone who faces life's challenges with courage and resilience. Visualize taking control of your own narrative, standing strong in your truth, and confronting obstacles with integrity and wisdom. This is the path of the Warrior, where personal responsibility leads to true empowerment.

Lena's Story: Logic Over Emotion and Fibromyalgia

Lena had always prided herself on her ability to remain calm under pressure. As a data analyst, her life revolved around logic and precision. Yet, when her father passed away and her long-term relationship ended, Lena buried her emotions, avoiding the overwhelming grief. She managed her life by focusing on the practical aspects, but the strain began to show.

Lena's story illustrates the **Computer shadow**—a shadow that relies on intellect while avoiding vulnerability. Instead of processing her feelings, Lena concentrated on controlling her environment, suppressing her emotions. This suppression eventually led to the development of fibromyalgia, where her body reflected the emotional tension she refused to confront.

The Conflict Shock (DHS)

Lena's emotional shock occurred when she received the unexpected news of her father's passing. Already emotionally detached from her recent breakup, this new grief triggered a **self-devaluation conflict**, manifesting through chronic fatigue and widespread pain. Her body, recognizing the unresolved emotional distress, responded by breaking down tissue, in alignment with German New Medicine's principles, trying to adapt to the unresolved emotional shock.

Hanging Healing and Cycles of Stress

Though Lena sought therapy to cope with her grief, her body remained in a **hanging healing** state—unable to fully heal as the emotional triggers kept reactivating the stress cycle. Her physical symptoms persisted because her emotional conflict had not fully resolved, and her body continued attempting to adapt. Fibromyalgia's pain and fatigue lingered as her body signalled that deeper emotional healing was needed.

Moving from Computer to Guru

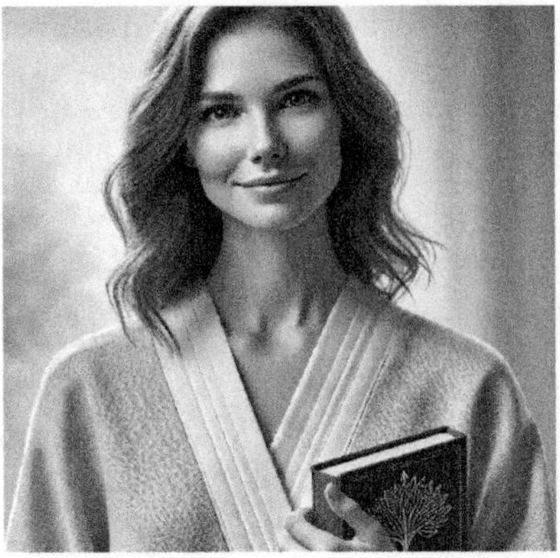

Lena's transformation from the **Computer** to the **Guru** archetype symbolizes her journey toward emotional integration. The Guru, unlike the Computer, embraces both intellect and intuition, recognizing that true wisdom comes from balancing logic with emotional depth.

The **Guru archetype** merges the analytical mind with the heart's emotional intelligence. As Lena began to trust her emotions and allow herself to feel vulnerable, she moved toward a more balanced way of living. The shift wasn't easy, but with each step, she learned that acknowledging and processing emotions didn't diminish her strength—it enhanced it.

Steps to Empowerment:

- **Acknowledge Your Emotions:** The Guru teaches us that suppressed emotions only deepen the conflict. Begin to acknowledge your emotions, even the uncomfortable ones, instead of burying them.
- **Balance Logic with Emotion:** Reflect on areas in your life where you rely too heavily on logic. How can you bring your emotions into the decision-making process?
- **Trust Your Intuition:** As the Guru learns, intuition and emotional intelligence are just as valuable as intellect. How can you learn to trust your inner wisdom more?

Visualize Your Transformation:

Imagine yourself as the empowered **Guru**—wise, connected, and emotionally aware. Envision the integration of your mind and heart, guiding you to navigate life's challenges with grace and insight. This is the path of the Guru, where intellect meets emotional depth, and true empowerment begins.

Clara's Story: Avoidance, Humour, and Fibromyalgia

Clara had always been the life of the party. Throwing herself into her social life, she used humour and distractions to avoid facing her deeper emotional struggles. Whether dealing with a failed relationship or stress at work, Clara kept herself busy, believing that as long as she was active, the emotional pain wouldn't catch up with her.

Clara's story illustrates the **Distractor shadow**, which evades difficult emotions by using humour or keeping busy. For Clara, her constant need to stay active was a way to avoid confronting the fear and grief beneath the surface. Over time, this avoidance manifested physically, triggering the widespread pain and fatigue of fibromyalgia—a condition rooted in unresolved self-devaluation conflicts.

The Conflict Shock (DHS)

The emotional shock came when Clara's mother suddenly fell ill. The event triggered a deep-seated **self-devaluation conflict**, as Clara felt inadequate in her caregiving role. The unresolved emotional turmoil led to widespread physical pain and chronic fatigue, as Clara's body responded to the unaddressed emotional strain.

Hanging Healing and Cycles of Stress

Though Clara sought therapy, her body remained in **hanging healing**—a state where the initial conflict was somewhat resolved, but recurring emotional triggers reactivated her symptoms. Her fibromyalgia persisted because the core emotional conflicts were not fully processed. Her body, following its biological programming, continued its attempts to heal while being interrupted by emotional stressors.

Moving from Distractor to Jester

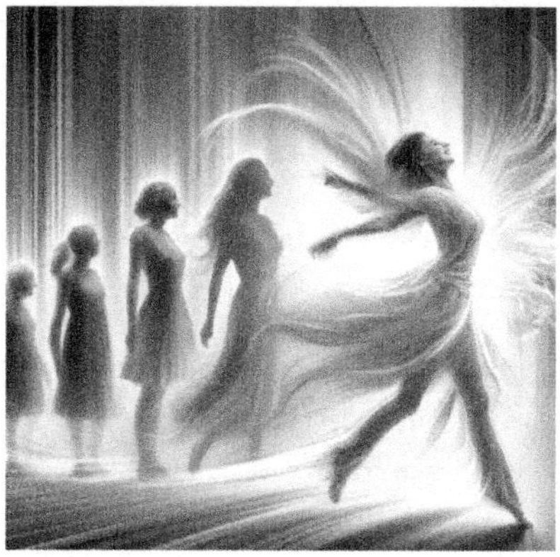

Clara's transformation from the Distractor to the **Jester archetype** marked the beginning of her true emotional healing. The Jester, the empowered version of the Distractor, uses humour as a way to heal and lighten difficult moments without avoiding emotions. For Clara, this shift meant using humour not as a shield but as a tool for self-awareness and healing.

The Jester archetype integrates both masculine energy—action and confrontation—and feminine energy—emotional expression and connection. Clara learned to embrace the Jester's playful energy to bring balance, facing her emotions while still using humour to bring perspective to life's challenges.

Steps to Empowerment:

- **Face Your Emotions:** Humour can be a powerful tool, but the Jester knows it's essential to confront the emotions behind the laughter. What emotions have you been avoiding? How can you begin to embrace and process them?
- **Use Humour Positively:** Explore how humour can lighten difficult situations without becoming a form of avoidance. How can you bring joy and emotional presence to your life?
- **Balance Playfulness with Presence:** The Jester knows how to balance joy with responsibility. How can you bring lightness into your life while staying emotionally grounded?

Visualize Your Transformation:

Imagine yourself as the **Jester**—someone who can bring joy to others while also staying emotionally grounded. Picture using humour to lighten tough situations, not as a way to escape but as a path to healing. This is the Jester's path, where playfulness meets presence, and humour aids in emotional healing.

Reflecting on the Stories: A Journey into the Emotional Landscape of Fibromyalgia

As we reflect on the stories of Sam, Rachel, Lena, and Clara, it's natural to wonder how these deeply personal experiences of emotional conflict may mirror your own life—or the lives of those you care about. Do any of these stories resonate with you? Have you or someone you know faced a traumatic loss, a profound sense of separation, or a significant conflict and yet not developed physical symptoms like those described? This begs a vital question: why do some individuals experience biological changes while others, despite similar conflicts, do not?

The Role of Conflict Resolution in Healing

It's crucial to understand that not everyone who experiences a **Conflict Shock (DHS)** will develop a condition like fibromyalgia. The body's response to emotional conflicts can vary. For some, the conflict is resolved quickly, consciously or unconsciously, allowing their body to heal without manifesting significant symptoms. Others may develop resilience or coping mechanisms over time that protect them from physical symptoms. The difference often lies in whether the emotional conflict is fully processed and resolved.

Why Do Some Develop Symptoms While Others Don't?

This introduces the concept of the **grey area**. You might have faced significant emotional conflicts without developing symptoms like chronic fatigue or pain—why? One reason could be that you resolved the conflict, perhaps without even realizing it. Another explanation is that over time, your personal growth and emotional awareness may have provided a protective buffer against biological responses, preventing the symptoms from manifesting.

Consider how people exposed to the same stressful situation or environment react differently. Some may develop symptoms of fibromyalgia, while others do not. The key lies in how each person processes the emotional experience. Those who resolve the conflict or have strong emotional and mental resources are often better equipped to avoid triggering the biological changes that result in fibromyalgia.

Building Resilience and Pre-emptive Healing

The stories of these women demonstrate what can happen when emotional conflicts go unresolved. However, they also offer hope. The fact that not everyone develops fibromyalgia or similar conditions after an emotional shock suggests that healing is possible—even after symptoms appear. By gaining a deeper understanding of our emotions, relationships, and inner conflicts, we can influence how we respond to life's challenges and potentially prevent or resolve physical symptoms.

A Better Way Forward

Throughout this book, we will explore various layers of emotional healing that can help prevent and resolve symptoms before they manifest physically. It's about more than just managing illness—it's about building resilience, fostering self-awareness, and using the tools available to resolve conflicts without triggering biological responses.

As you continue reading, reflect on your own emotional landscape. What conflicts have you faced, and have they been fully resolved? How can you better prepare yourself emotionally for future challenges, ensuring that both your mind and body remain in balance?

This book offers not just solutions but hope and empowerment. By integrating the body, mind, and emotions, you can embrace a path toward true wellness and recovery. Keep an open mind as we delve deeper into these concepts and remember—healing is possible.

Introduction

If you're reading this book, it's likely that you or someone you care about is facing the complex and often misunderstood challenge of fibromyalgia. Persistent symptoms like muscle pain, fatigue, and sensitivity can feel isolating, especially when conventional medicine may not seem to address the root causes or provide lasting relief.

Perhaps you're searching for a deeper understanding of why these symptoms arise—something beyond simply managing them. This book offers an alternative view, exploring how emotions, stress, and unresolved conflicts are tied to your health through the lens of German New Medicine (GNM) and integrative healing approaches.

Reach out for help.

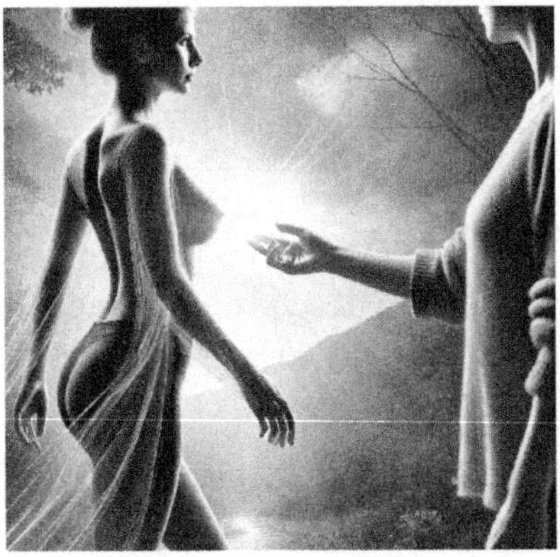

A Journey Towards True Healing and Empowerment

Imagine breaking free from the fear and uncertainty that often accompany chronic conditions like fibromyalgia. Picture waking each day with a sense of empowerment, armed with tools and understanding to reclaim your health. Healing goes beyond managing symptoms; it's about uncovering and addressing long-buried conflicts and emotions to unlock profound transformation.

This book invites you into a deeper exploration of the powerful connections between your mind, body, and spirit. You'll discover that healing isn't something that passively happens to you; it's a process you actively participate in by understanding how your thoughts, beliefs, and emotions shape your physical well-being.

You might wonder, "Can I truly influence my health in such a profound way?" The answer is yes. Embracing a new perspective is a vital first step, opening you to the possibility that your health challenges can serve as guides toward personal growth and transformation.

Throughout this book, we'll uncover how unresolved conflicts, unexpressed emotions, and limiting beliefs can manifest as physical symptoms, specifically those associated with fibromyalgia. You'll learn to identify these hidden influences, and, through practical strategies and insights, align your mind, body, and spirit for a life filled with vitality and wellness.

This journey requires courage, but by picking up this book, you've already taken the first step. Now, let's go deeper together—to explore the roots of your health challenges and reclaim the joy and vitality that are rightfully yours.

Why This Book?

Years of working with clients have shown me that conventional methods often fall short of truly resolving health challenges like fibromyalgia. My approach combines the insights of German New Medicine (GNM), META-Health, and Strategic Intervention to illuminate how emotional conflicts can lead to biological changes we identify as disease. I have witnessed incredible transformations when clients embraced the mind-body connection and took ownership of their healing journeys.

This book is part of a series that tackles specific health conditions, each exploring the principles of GNM and the profound effect of emotional healing on physical symptoms. For an even broader perspective, consider my first book, *The Human Reboot: Demystifying Disease*, which offers a comprehensive look at the mind-body connection.

As we explore these ideas, remember: true healing involves more than just treating symptoms. It's about understanding the inner patterns and conflicts that may be influencing your health and empowering yourself to work with your body's natural processes. This journey invites you to see your health not as a static state but as an evolving relationship between your mind, body, and spirit. Together, we'll explore how to align these elements for the fullest expression of wellness.

The Intersection of Belief, Spirituality, and Disease

A diagnosis related to fibromyalgia can be life-altering, challenging both belief systems and understandings of health. Many grapple with questions like, "Why is this happening to me?" or "What purpose does this pain serve?" From a religious perspective, this might feel like a test, while others view it as an unfortunate randomness. But what if fibromyalgia were neither punishment nor random? What if it were part of a meaningful biological response rooted in our natural instincts?

This view is central to German New Medicine (GNM) and META-Health. According to Dr. Ryke Geerd Hamer, diseases aren't accidental malfunctions but purposeful biological adaptations designed to help the body cope with deep emotional conflicts. In GNM, disease is seen as a biological survival program triggered by an emotional shock. For those dealing with fibromyalgia, unresolved conflicts—often linked to self-worth, feeling overwhelmed, or chronic emotional stress—can manifest as prolonged pain and fatigue.

This perspective can be spiritually comforting. For people of faith, it suggests that suffering isn't meaningless, but rather a pathway for growth and healing. For those without spiritual beliefs, it offers a framework showing that physical symptoms are the body's way of signalling unresolved emotional conflicts rather than arbitrary occurrences. In both cases, the GNM approach transforms the view of disease from one of fear to one of understanding, where symptoms become a guide to healing the inner self.

The Human Condition

When facing fibromyalgia or chronic pain, questions about life, purpose, and beliefs often surface. It's common to wonder, "Why is this happening to me?" For some, this may challenge their spiritual beliefs, while others without a particular faith may feel that life has dealt them an unfair hand. But what if fibromyalgia was not a flaw in the body, but a biologically meaningful response to deep-seated emotional stress and unresolved inner conflicts?

In German New Medicine (GNM), Dr. Ryke Geerd Hamer's research suggested that symptoms like pain, fatigue, and inflammation can be responses to unresolved emotional conflicts. Dr. Hamer observed that conditions such as fibromyalgia emerge not from random defects but as a way the body adapts to cope with deeply rooted psychological stress. He found that chronic symptoms, rather than being senseless, are the body's attempts to heal in response to significant shocks or stresses. For people dealing with fibromyalgia, these stressors often relate to self-worth, feelings of overwhelm, and the repeated suppression of personal needs.

For those with a spiritual outlook, GNM's perspective offers hope: illness is not a punishment but a pathway to healing. By understanding fibromyalgia as the body's response to internal conflict, patients can move from feeling at odds with their bodies to seeing their symptoms as part of a natural, if uncomfortable, healing process. This view allows them to approach fibromyalgia as an opportunity for emotional growth and resolution rather than simply a battle against pain.

The Role of Modern Medicine

Modern medicine has made impressive advancements in managing acute crises and performing life-saving interventions. Yet, when it comes to chronic conditions like fibromyalgia, conventional approaches may sometimes fall short, as they tend to focus on managing symptoms rather than resolving underlying causes.

In many traditional medical frameworks, chronic pain or fatigue is often viewed as a malfunction of the body. Patients are frequently prescribed medications that can alleviate discomfort temporarily but don't address the root emotional and psychological stressors that GNM identifies as primary triggers. German New Medicine proposes that symptoms like those in fibromyalgia are not signs of a failing body but part of the body's effort to resolve unresolved emotional conflicts and trauma.

It's essential to recognize that while pharmaceuticals provide necessary relief, they may not be the complete solution for long-term wellness. Instead of merely managing symptoms, GNM offers an approach that sees fibromyalgia as an opportunity to address deeper emotional patterns and resolve the biological programs keeping the body in a cycle of "hanging healing." This perspective allows individuals to view their condition not as an unending struggle but as a guide to identify, address, and heal long-held conflicts.

In this view, modern medicine and GNM can complement one another. Modern treatments provide necessary support and relief, while GNM's insights help patients understand and work through the root causes of their pain. By integrating these approaches, those with fibromyalgia can achieve a fuller, more meaningful journey toward lasting health.

German New Medicine: A New Understanding of Health

German New Medicine (GNM) was pioneered by Dr. Ryke Geerd Hamer in the late 1970s after he experienced a profound loss—the tragic death of his son, Dirk. Shortly after, Dr. Hamer himself was diagnosed with testicular cancer, leading him to wonder if this emotional shock had contributed to his illness. His search for answers resulted in years of research, uncovering links between emotional trauma and physical disease, forming the foundation of GNM.

GNM introduces a revolutionary view of disease. Rather than seeing illness as a malfunction, GNM asserts that disease is an adaptive biological response to emotional conflicts. These emotional shocks, or conflict shocks (DHS), influence the mind, brain, and specific tissues or organs, initiating a biological adaptation intended to help the body cope with trauma.

In the context of fibromyalgia, GNM explores how self-devaluation conflicts—feelings of inadequacy, burden, or overwhelm—can contribute to symptoms like chronic pain, fatigue, and muscle stiffness. When we experience an internalized sense of low self-worth, particularly when "everything else is put before us," the body may activate a biological response, breaking down and attempting to rebuild tissues to adapt to this devaluation. This response is an attempt to strengthen areas of the body in response to perceived inadequacy, but when the conflict remains unresolved, it can lead to ongoing cycles of pain and fatigue, known in GNM as "hanging healing."

Through GNM, we gain insight into how our body's responses are not arbitrary failures but are meaningful, adaptive processes aimed at helping us survive emotional trauma. Dr. Hamer's research identified the Five Biological Laws, which describe how these adaptations progress. These laws apply to all life forms and offer a framework for understanding illness not as an error but as part of a survival-based biological response.

Understanding these connections provides a new lens for approaching fibromyalgia. By addressing and resolving underlying emotional conflicts, individuals may allow the body to complete its healing cycle naturally. GNM emphasizes that these adaptations are not flaws but rather biologically purposeful responses designed to help us manage and ultimately heal from unresolved emotional stresses.

The Five Biological Laws of German New Medicine

At the heart of German New Medicine (GNM) lies Dr. Ryke Geerd Hamer's groundbreaking discovery of the Five Biological Laws, offering a transformative perspective on the origins of disease. These laws are universal, applying to all living beings, and they provide a structured approach to understanding how emotional conflicts trigger specific biological programs in the body.

Rather than viewing disease as a failure or error, GNM teaches that illness is an adaptive, intelligent response designed to help the body endure unexpected emotional shocks. These emotional conflicts not only impact the psyche but also influence the brain and corresponding organs or tissues, initiating a biologically purposeful response aimed at supporting the individual through the conflict.

For those dealing with chronic conditions like fibromyalgia, the Five Biological Laws present a holistic way of understanding the link between emotions, the brain, and the body. By viewing the symptoms of fibromyalgia—such as pain, fatigue, and muscle stiffness—through the GNM lens, we can explore how unresolved self-devaluation conflicts and other hidden emotional triggers contribute to these chronic experiences. Understanding these laws allows us to harmonize with the body's natural healing processes, rather than working against them.

Let's now explore each of the Five Biological Laws in detail, uncovering how unresolved emotional conflicts may contribute to the chronic symptoms seen in fibromyalgia and how they represent a meaningful biological response.

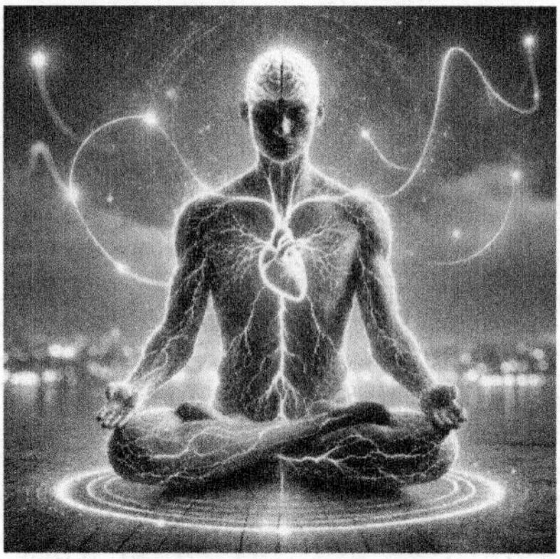

1. The Iron Rule of Cancer (The First Biological Law)

The First Biological Law, known as the Iron Rule of Disease, proposes that every condition, including fibromyalgia, begins with a DHS (Dirk Hamer Syndrome)—an intense, unexpected emotional shock that feels isolating and profoundly stressful. This event impacts the psyche, the brain, and a specific organ or tissue in the body, creating a ripple effect:

The Psyche: The person experiences an intense emotional conflict, often tied to self-devaluation themes like feeling unworthy or underappreciated, leading to deep psychological stress.

The Brain: This conflict registers as a Hamer Focus (HH) in a specific area of the brain. This impact appears on a scan as concentric rings in a region linked to the affected tissue.

The Organ/Tissue: The organ or tissue governed by the impacted brain region reacts accordingly. In fibromyalgia, muscles, nerves, and connective tissues are affected, often reflecting long-standing self-doubt or feeling undervalued. The biological response results in physical tension, pain, or fatigue as the body responds to the stress embedded in these tissues.

For the DHS to initiate this response, three specific criteria are necessary:

Unexpected: The emotional shock catches the individual off guard.

Dramatic: The conflict holds a significant emotional impact.

Isolating: The person feels unsupported or unable to express their inner conflict.

In fibromyalgia, the themes often involve *self-devaluation conflicts*—chronic self-doubt, feelings of worthlessness, or long periods of feeling unappreciated.

These conflicts place stress on muscles and connective tissues, contributing to the familiar strain, tension, and fatigue experienced in fibromyalgia.

Recap for the First Biological Law: According to the First Biological Law, conditions like fibromyalgia stem from an intense emotional shock that the individual struggles to process. This shock affects the mind, brain, and specific body tissues simultaneously. By recognizing these root conflicts—often tied to self-worth and self-value—those with fibromyalgia can work towards resolving underlying emotional tensions, initiating the body's natural healing process.

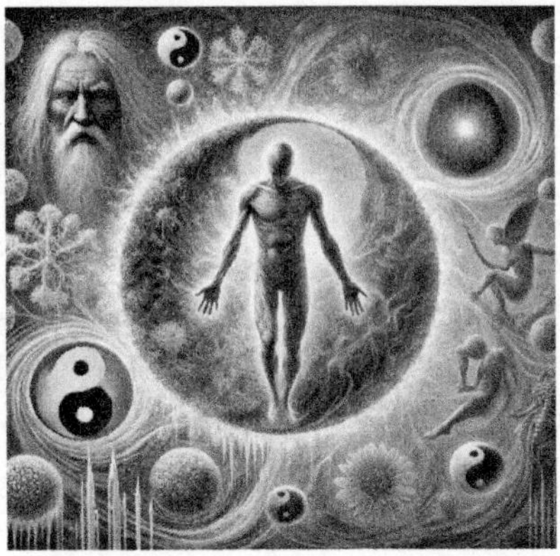

2. The Law of Two Phases (The Second Biological Law)

The Second Biological Law explains that every condition progresses through two distinct phases: the conflict-active phase and the healing phase, provided that the underlying emotional conflict is resolved.

Conflict-Active Phase: In the conflict-active phase, an unresolved emotional conflict keeps the individual in a heightened state of stress, governed by the sympathetic nervous system (responsible for "fight-or-flight" responses). The body displays signs of increased alertness, energy conservation, and readiness to react to perceived threats. Some common physical indicators include:

Cold hands and feet

Loss of appetite

Difficulty sleeping and persistent mental alertness

In fibromyalgia, self-devaluation conflicts—often involving feelings of inadequacy, failure, or lack of support—can lead to chronic tension in muscles and tissues. This tension is not arbitrary but a biologically driven response designed to cope with the stress of unresolved self-worth conflicts. Over time, however, it can result in muscle tightness or even tissue degeneration, contributing to pain and discomfort.

Healing Phase: Once the conflict is resolved, whether through emotional release, conflict resolution, or a change in circumstances, the body transitions to the healing phase. This phase is characterized by parasympathetic dominance ("rest-and-digest" mode), where the body begins to repair and restore balance. During the healing phase, symptoms may include:

Inflammation and swelling

Increased pain and sensitivity

Fatigue and a heightened awareness of discomfort

In the context of fibromyalgia, the healing phase is when muscle soreness, stiffness, and fatigue are often most pronounced. These symptoms can be misinterpreted as signs of a "flare-up" or disease progression, but in reality, they indicate the body's attempt to repair tissues and recover from the effects of the prolonged stress phase. This law challenges the view of symptoms as "illness" and encourages us to see them as part of the body's natural process of healing and rebalancing.

Chronic Conditions: Unresolved or frequently re-triggered conflicts can lead to a back-and-forth between the active and healing phases, creating a cycle of chronic symptoms. In fibromyalgia, if self-devaluation conflicts remain unaddressed or recur due to environmental triggers or unresolved emotional patterns, the body may be stuck in this cycle indefinitely. This prolonged cycle explains why individuals with fibromyalgia experience ongoing pain, fatigue, and sensitivity—symptoms that reflect an attempt by the body to reach resolution and restore balance.

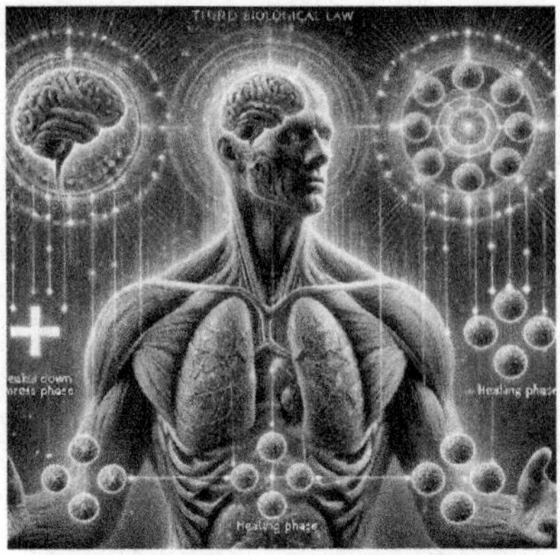

3. The Ontogenetic System of Tumours (The Third Biological Law)

Before We Dive into the Third Biological Law

Imagine the Earth billions of years ago, at a time when life was just beginning. Early organisms, floating in primordial oceans, were focused solely on survival. These simple organisms absorbed nutrients, protected themselves from their environment, and reproduced with an uncomplicated biological system. Over time, as life evolved, so did the complexity of these systems, ultimately giving rise to three primary tissue layers within all multicellular organisms: the endoderm, mesoderm, and ectoderm. Each layer evolved to handle specific survival functions—nourishment, protection, and connection.

The Endoderm: The Foundation for Survival
The first tissue layer, the endoderm, governs essential functions like digestion and respiration, laying the groundwork for survival by ensuring the intake of nutrients and oxygen. Imagine a primitive organism absorbing nutrients from its surroundings—its sole focus is on obtaining the resources needed to survive.

The Mesoderm: The Armor and Movement Layer
As life forms became more advanced, they needed mechanisms for defence, mobility, and structural support. The mesoderm evolved to create muscles, bones, and connective tissues, which protect and enable movement, allowing organisms to adapt to threats and explore their surroundings.

The Ectoderm: The Interface with the External World
With further complexity, the ectoderm developed to support sensory perception, communication, and social connection. This layer includes the skin, sensory organs, and nervous system, allowing organisms to sense

changes in their environment, communicate, and build relationships vital to survival.

These three layers—endoderm, mesoderm, and ectoderm—form the biological foundation of our bodies. They represent evolutionary solutions for handling the physical and emotional challenges of survival, each governed by specific regions of the brain.

The Ontogenetic System of Tumours and Tissue Changes

The Third Biological Law of German New Medicine (GNM) explains that the type of biological response (such as cell growth, tissue loss, or functional change) is determined by the tissue's embryological origin. The three tissue layers—endoderm, mesoderm, and ectoderm—are controlled by different brain regions and respond to distinct types of emotional conflicts. This understanding is essential in fibromyalgia, where symptoms like muscle pain, fatigue, and sensitivity are the body's responses to unresolved emotional conflicts.

Biological Responses by Tissue Layer in Fibromyalgia

Endoderm (Controlled by the Brainstem)
The endoderm governs tissues involved in basic survival functions, such as glands and parts of the digestive and respiratory systems. This layer is particularly responsive to conflicts tied to survival, nurturing, and protection.

Conflict-Active Phase: During this phase, an unresolved nurturing or self-preservation conflict may lead to cell proliferation in endodermal tissues. For instance, digestive issues might arise as the body tries to increase its capacity for nourishment during times of perceived threat.

Healing Phase: Once the conflict is resolved, the body initiates a repair process. Microorganisms such as bacteria often assist in breaking down excess tissue, helping restore balance. In fibromyalgia, this can manifest as inflammation, swelling, or tenderness, signalling the body's attempt to process and release deeply held emotional stress.

Mesoderm (Controlled by the Cerebellum and Cerebral Medulla)
Mesodermal tissues, which include muscles, bones, and connective tissues,

handle self-protection and self-worth conflicts. They are divided into two subtypes based on brain control:

Old Mesoderm (Cerebellum): This tissue group, which includes the body's protective layers, reacts to defensive conflicts, such as feeling vulnerable or under threat. In fibromyalgia, old mesodermal tissues may become tense or thicken in response to perceived external dangers, leading to chronic muscle tension.

New Mesoderm (Cerebral Medulla): This group includes skeletal muscles and tissues that respond to self-devaluation conflicts—feelings of inadequacy, failure, or being unworthy. In fibromyalgia, unresolved self-devaluation may cause tissue degradation or muscle atrophy in the conflict-active phase. Once healing begins, the body focuses on tissue rebuilding, often resulting in symptoms like pain, stiffness, and fatigue as it attempts to regain strength and balance.

Ectoderm (Controlled by the Cerebral Cortex)
The ectoderm layer includes tissues involved in sensory perception, connection, and communication, such as the skin, sensory pathways, and mucous membranes. Conflicts here often involve feelings of separation or emotional disconnection.

Conflict-Active Phase: In this phase, separation conflicts may cause cell loss in ectodermal tissues, leading to sensations of heightened pain sensitivity or discomfort. In fibromyalgia, this is reflected in increased pain perception and discomfort, which may feel overwhelming and isolating.

Healing Phase: As the conflict resolves, ectodermal tissues regenerate, often accompanied by temporary swelling, pain, or heightened sensitivity. These symptoms can manifest as flare-ups in fibromyalgia, where the body intensifies its healing process and brings unresolved emotional experiences to the surface.

Implications of the Third Biological Law for Fibromyalgia

The Third Biological Law reveals that our bodies respond to conflicts in organized, specific ways, shaped by evolutionary adaptations. Tissues respond based on their embryological origins and brain connections, each having a unique reaction to different types of emotional conflicts. In fibromyalgia, this understanding suggests that symptoms like muscle pain, fatigue, and sensitivity are part of the body's effort to adapt to unresolved emotional stresses, whether they are nurturing conflicts, self-devaluation, or separation issues.

This perspective empowers individuals with fibromyalgia to view their bodies not as malfunctioning but as biologically programmed for survival. Through GNM, we understand that chronic pain and fatigue are not random but part of the body's sophisticated response to help us cope with and process deep emotional conflicts.

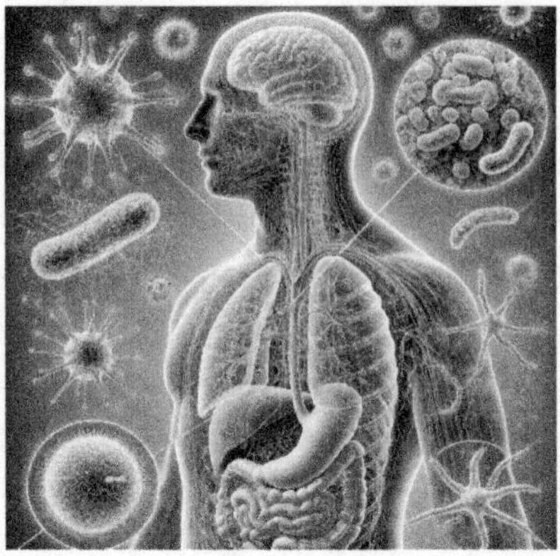

4. The Role of Microbes in the Healing Phase (The Fourth Biological Law)

The Fourth Biological Law of German New Medicine (GNM) offers a revolutionary view of microbes—bacteria, fungi, and viruses—seeing them as essential allies in the healing process rather than harmful invaders. In GNM, microbes are not the cause of disease but rather assist the body in the recovery phase once an emotional conflict is resolved.

How Microbes Aid in Healing

Each type of microbe has a specific function during the healing phase, depending on the tissue type and the nature of the conflict:

Bacteria and Fungi: These microbes help break down and remove excess cells that may have accumulated during the conflict-active phase. For example, if tissues grew or swelled due to stress or tension, bacteria and fungi assist in breaking down these excess cells, allowing the body to return to balance.

Viruses: In cases where cell loss occurred during the conflict, viruses support the regeneration of tissues. They are particularly helpful in restoring areas where deterioration or damage has occurred, contributing to cellular repair.

Microbes in the Context of Fibromyalgia

In fibromyalgia, where chronic muscle pain, fatigue, and connective tissue issues often result from unresolved self-devaluation conflicts, microbes play a significant role in the body's healing cycle:

Muscle and Connective Tissue Recovery: For instance, if there has been prolonged stress affecting muscles and connective tissues, bacteria may be involved in reducing inflammation and breaking down any overbuilt tissue. This aligns with the body's effort to release stored tension and repair strained muscles.

Tissue Regeneration: In cases where prolonged stress or self-devaluation has led to tissue degradation or muscle fatigue, viruses and other microbes assist in tissue regeneration, facilitating the body's natural recovery.

The Brain's Role in Microbe Activation

Dr. Hamer observed that the brain controls and activates microbes precisely when the body enters the healing phase. This activation aligns with the type of tissue involved and the stage of recovery:

Endodermal Tissues (e.g., parts of the digestive system, certain glands, controlled by the brainstem): In these tissues, fungi and bacteria help break down excess cells that accumulated during the active conflict. This can be relevant to fibromyalgia if digestive issues are involved, as bacteria may assist in rebalancing gut health as part of the overall healing process.

Mesodermal Tissues (e.g., muscles, bones, connective tissues, controlled by the cerebral medulla and cerebellum): Mesodermal tissues, which are heavily involved in fibromyalgia, use bacteria to repair and restore cells affected by degradation or tension. The body's reliance on microbes for muscle and connective tissue repair underscores the adaptive response to chronic emotional conflicts like self-devaluation.

Ectodermal Tissues (e.g., skin, nerves, sensory organs, controlled by the cerebral cortex): These tissues engage viruses and other microbes to aid in the regeneration process after a separation conflict or emotional stress. In fibromyalgia, heightened pain sensitivity and nerve issues may be part of this healing phase, where microbes assist in restoring normal sensory function.

Implications of the Fourth Biological Law in Fibromyalgia

The Fourth Biological Law highlights that microbes are not enemies but rather supportive participants in the body's recovery process. This understanding reframes our perception of microbes, showing that bacteria, fungi, and viruses assist the body in restoring balance, reducing inflammation, and aiding in tissue repair once emotional conflicts are addressed.

In fibromyalgia, symptoms like pain, inflammation, and heightened sensitivity are part of the body's effort to heal. Recognizing the role of microbes can help individuals view these symptoms not as signs of disease but as evidence of the body's natural recovery processes. Understanding this allows individuals to approach healing with a more harmonious perspective, knowing that the body is designed to use these organisms in its journey toward balance and resilience.

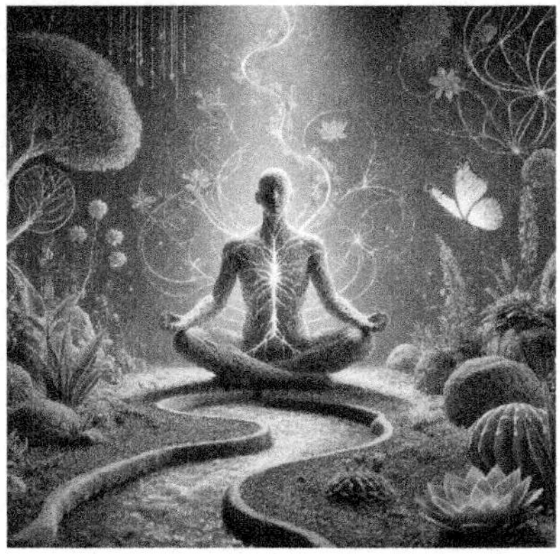

5. The Quintessence (The Fifth Biological Law)

The Fifth Biological Law, also known as the Quintessence, reveals a fundamental truth about disease: that all conditions, including chronic illnesses like fibromyalgia, are not malfunctions but rather part of Special Biological Programs (SBS) designed by evolution to support survival. This perspective transforms our understanding of disease from a random error to a purposeful, adaptive response.

According to the Quintessence, every symptom—whether it be cell growth, cell loss, or functional changes—serves a biological purpose, helping the body cope with unresolved emotional conflicts. Diseases are not arbitrary; they are intentional responses, signalling to the individual that there is a deeper emotional or psychological issue needing resolution.

The Quintessence in the Context of Fibromyalgia

For those experiencing fibromyalgia, symptoms like persistent pain, fatigue, and inflammation are the body's responses to unresolved emotional conflicts, particularly self-devaluation and prolonged stress. According to this law, these symptoms are not meaningless but are biologically meaningful adaptations, designed to help the body manage internalized conflicts.

In fibromyalgia, every element of the condition has a purpose shaped by the body's instinct to survive and adapt:

Pain Sensitivity: Heightened pain sensitivity may represent an alert system, encouraging individuals to address lingering emotional stressors. It's as if the body is amplifying sensations to signal that something unresolved is demanding attention.

Muscle Fatigue: Chronic fatigue and muscle weakness reflect the body's attempt to conserve energy and slow down, a common reaction in response to prolonged stress or feelings of inadequacy. By limiting physical output, the body encourages rest and introspection, giving the individual a chance to confront underlying emotional conflicts.

Inflammation: Inflammatory responses in fibromyalgia signify the body's efforts to protect and repair. In GNM, inflammation is often associated with the healing phase, meaning the body is actively working on resolving and restoring areas impacted by emotional stress.

Embracing the Purpose of Symptoms

Understanding the Quintessence allows us to see fibromyalgia symptoms not as signs of failure but as meaningful reactions meant to aid survival. These symptoms push us to pause, reflect, and address unresolved emotional challenges that may have been overlooked or suppressed. When we acknowledge these signals, we open ourselves to the possibility of true healing by addressing the emotional roots of our physical condition.

Conclusion: The Power of German New Medicine

The Five Biological Laws of German New Medicine provide a revolutionary framework for understanding health, especially in the context of chronic conditions like fibromyalgia. They demonstrate that diseases are not random malfunctions but biologically meaningful programs activated by unresolved emotional conflicts.

By identifying and resolving these conflicts, we unlock the potential for healing on the deepest levels—physically, emotionally, and mentally. Embracing this perspective allows us to work with our bodies rather than against them, utilizing the natural intelligence of our biological systems to move toward profound healing and well-being.

The Three Exceptions: Physical Trauma, Toxicity, and Deficiency

While **German New Medicine (GNM)** primarily focuses on unresolved **emotional conflicts** as the root cause of disease, there are three important exceptions where **physical factors** also play a critical role in health. These exceptions—**physical trauma**, **toxicity**, and **deficiency**—must be considered, as they can impact the body's ability to heal and maintain balance. Addressing these factors alongside emotional healing is essential for a complete and holistic approach to well-being.

1. Physical Trauma

Physical trauma, such as injury or surgery, directly affects the body's tissues, disrupting the natural balance. Unlike emotional conflicts, which initiate biological programs on a deeper level, physical trauma requires targeted care to support the body's recovery. Adequate **nutrition** plays a key role in this healing process, providing the body with essential building blocks like **protein**, **collagen**, and **healthy fats** to repair damaged tissue.

2. Toxicity

Toxicity refers to harmful substances in the body, but it also encompasses **mental toxicity**—the negative thoughts and beliefs that can have a damaging effect on health. In GNM, emotional conflicts play a central role in disease, but physical and mental toxicity must not be overlooked.

- **Physical Toxicity**: Exposure to **chemicals**, **pollutants**, and **processed foods** can overwhelm the body's natural detoxification systems. This might include environmental toxins, unhealthy diets, or prolonged exposure to harmful substances, which impair the body's ability to heal.
- **Mental Toxicity**: **Negative beliefs** or **chronic stress** can act as toxic agents on the mind, manifesting as emotional conflicts that impact physical health. Toxic thoughts like self-criticism or the fear of judgment can perpetuate emotional stress, contributing to the development of symptoms.

3. Deficiency

Deficiency refers not only to the lack of essential nutrients but also to a deficiency of **reliable information** and strategies needed for healing and growth. Both forms of deficiency—physical and intellectual—can hinder the body's ability to achieve balance.

- **Nutritional Deficiency**: The body requires a variety of **vitamins**, **minerals**, and **nutrients** to support its healing process. A deficiency in these nutrients can impede recovery and make the body more vulnerable to disease.

- **Deficiency of Information**: In today's world, access to accurate, **proven strategies** for health can be difficult to find. The abundance of misinformation can prevent individuals from making informed choices about their health, leaving them without the guidance necessary for true healing.

By considering these three exceptions—**physical trauma**, **toxicity**, and **deficiency**—alongside the emotional aspects of disease, a more comprehensive and integrative approach to healing can be achieved. For individuals facing **Fibromyalgia** or other health challenges, addressing these factors in tandem with emotional healing allows for a deeper, more sustainable return to balance and wellness.

Overview of Fibromyalgia and Its Emotional Roots

Fibromyalgia, characterized by widespread pain, fatigue, and emotional strain. In GNM, fibromyalgia symptoms are viewed as biologically meaningful responses to unresolved emotional conflicts or life stresses that remain active, causing a "hanging healing" state. This process can generate a cycle of symptoms, as the body attempts to resolve conflicts related to self-worth, social support, or resilience in facing long-standing difficulties.

Emotional Conflict Themes Related to Fibromyalgia
GNM suggests that fibromyalgia symptoms may result from recurring, unresolved conflicts tied to one's sense of self, personal resilience, and relationships. For example:

1. **Self-Devaluation Conflict**
    - *Nature of Conflict*: This conflict occurs when individuals feel inadequate or inferior, possibly due to challenging life situations or chronic stress. It's common in those experiencing long-term struggles, such as with work-life balance or caregiving.
    - *Biological Response*: In cases of self-devaluation, tissues related to the musculoskeletal system may be impacted, resulting in the muscular pain and joint stiffness often seen in fibromyalgia. The body's response is an attempt to strengthen and adapt to perceived weakness.
2. **Isolation Conflict**
    - *Nature of Conflict*: Isolation conflicts are associated with feeling emotionally or socially disconnected, possibly triggered by relationship breakdowns, loss, or significant life transitions that leave individuals feeling unsupported.
    - *Biological Response*: Feelings of loneliness or abandonment may impact the nervous system, contributing to sensations of widespread pain and fatigue, which are hallmark symptoms of fibromyalgia. The nervous system's hypersensitivity may represent the body's adaptation to perceived emotional vulnerability.

3. **Endurance or Resilience Conflict**
    - *Nature of Conflict*: Many people with fibromyalgia have faced long-term stress, financial strain, or persistent relationship challenges. They may feel overwhelmed by the need to "keep going" despite exhaustion.
    - *Biological Response*: The body might adapt by creating heightened nervous system sensitivity, leading to chronic fatigue and the sleep disturbances common in fibromyalgia.

Conditions and Symptoms: How Emotional Conflicts Manifest in Fibromyalgia

1. **Muscle Pain and Stiffness (Self-Devaluation Conflict)**
    - *Emotional Conflict*: Persistent feelings of inadequacy, often stemming from self-criticism or perceived failure, are common in fibromyalgia. This conflict may be reinforced by demanding life circumstances or personal expectations.
    - *Biological Response*: The body's response may manifest as musculoskeletal pain, reflecting an attempt to strengthen the areas affected by perceived weakness. Symptoms may worsen in the healing phase, with pain intensifying as the body seeks resolution.
2. **Chronic Fatigue (Endurance Conflict)**
    - *Emotional Conflict*: Long-term stress and resilience-based conflicts can result in fatigue, reflecting the body's attempt to conserve energy under ongoing pressure.
    - *Biological Response*: The constant state of perceived demand on resilience can lead to fatigue, disrupted sleep, and cognitive fog, manifesting as "fibro fog" and profound tiredness.
3. **Hypersensitivity to Pain (Isolation or Abandonment Conflict)**
    - *Emotional Conflict*: Feelings of abandonment or social isolation contribute to a heightened pain response, as the body interprets isolation as a need for heightened vigilance.

- *Biological Response*: This state can lead to heightened pain perception and a chronic sense of bodily discomfort, where everyday activities seem more strenuous due to this hypersensitivity.

Integrating Modern Medical Perspectives and GNM for Fibromyalgia

Modern Medical Perspective

While GNM provides a unique understanding of fibromyalgia through the lens of emotional conflicts, conventional medicine approaches fibromyalgia as a disorder of pain processing in the nervous system, often treated with medications, cognitive therapy, and physical rehabilitation.

1. **Causes and Tissue Responses**
   - *Conventional View*: Fibromyalgia is often explained by genetics, sleep disorders, or imbalances in pain-regulating neurotransmitters. Traditional treatments address pain reduction, muscle relaxation, and improved sleep.
   - *GNM View*: GNM attributes the body's chronic pain and fatigue in fibromyalgia to ongoing emotional conflicts, suggesting that resolution of these conflicts can naturally reduce the need for medication.
2. **Treatment Approaches**
   - *Conventional Treatment*: Pain management, stress reduction, and physical therapy are core components of fibromyalgia treatment. Antidepressants and medications for sleep and anxiety may also be prescribed.
   - *GNM Approach*: GNM emphasizes identifying and resolving emotional conflicts, with support for self-awareness and emotional resilience. Physical interventions remain supportive, rather than primary, to aid the body's natural adaptation.

Conclusion: Embracing a German New Medicine Approach to Fibromyalgia

Adopting a GNM-informed perspective encourages individuals with fibromyalgia to explore unresolved emotional conflicts as part of their path to healing. Rather than viewing fibromyalgia as an incurable, lifelong condition, GNM invites a holistic understanding that treats symptoms as adaptive responses. Resolving emotional conflicts may help break the cycle of chronic pain and fatigue, allowing a path forward that integrates both physical and emotional healing.

Understanding the Role of Emotional Conflicts and Significant Events

Before we explore the Six Human Needs, let's pause to remember an important point: while many chronic conditions, including fibromyalgia, may be linked to unresolved emotional conflicts, there are exceptions to this rule. Physical trauma, toxicity, and nutrient deficiency can also impact the body independently of emotional health, influencing recovery and resilience.

In German New Medicine (GNM), it's emphasized that the biological programs leading to symptoms such as chronic pain and fatigue are not triggered by minor emotional stresses or everyday frustrations. Instead, they're initiated by intense, unexpected traumatic events that produce deep emotional shocks—what GNM refers to as a DHS (Dirk Hamer Syndrome).

While fulfilling our needs in unproductive ways can create ongoing stress or dissatisfaction, it's important to note that this alone does not typically lead to biological responses like fibromyalgia symptoms. The purpose of exploring the Six Human Needs is to build emotional resilience, preparing us to respond more effectively if a DHS occurs, reducing the risk of triggering fibromyalgia symptoms or similar chronic conditions.

Proactive Emotional Health: Reducing Biological Conflict Triggers

Recognizing how we meet our needs allows us to proactively manage emotional stress and build resilience for future conflicts. This isn't about avoiding negative emotions or behaviors but about cultivating emotional balance and self-awareness. By doing so, if a significant, unexpected event arises, we are better equipped to manage it without triggering the biological responses associated with fibromyalgia, such as chronic muscle tension, pain, and fatigue.

In summary, while living by the shadow self or meeting needs in unproductive ways doesn't directly cause conditions like fibromyalgia, understanding and addressing these patterns equips us to handle impactful life events without overwhelming the body's biological systems. This approach helps reduce fear, improves emotional health, and strengthens overall resilience.

The Body's Healing Capacity: Moving Beyond Chronic Pain

It's clear that significant emotional conflicts can trigger biological responses, yet the body also has a remarkable capacity to heal once these conflicts are resolved. Just as unresolved emotional conflicts can contribute to chronic conditions like fibromyalgia, resolving these conflicts can prompt the body to begin healing, sometimes in ways that seem unexpected or even miraculous.

This phenomenon, often perceived as spontaneous recovery, is understood in GNM as a natural biological process. Dr. Ryke Geerd Hamer discovered this connection after experiencing the traumatic loss of his son, which led to his own health crisis. He realized that his physical symptoms were linked to emotional trauma, revealing the deeper ties between unresolved emotional conflicts and chronic health issues.

Similarly, in fibromyalgia, recovery can begin when the emotional conflicts triggering chronic pain and fatigue are resolved. This insight highlights the body's natural healing potential and points to ways we can engage in proactive emotional health for lasting well-being.

Spontaneous Remission: Demystifying a Natural Phenomenon in Fibromyalgia

Spontaneous remission has often been viewed as a miraculous or unexplainable recovery from chronic and complex conditions like fibromyalgia. However, from the perspective of German New Medicine (GNM), this phenomenon can be understood as a natural and meaningful part of the body's biological response. Dr. Ryke Geerd Hamer, the founder of GNM, discovered this connection after his own diagnosis of testicular cancer, which occurred following the tragic loss of his son. This personal experience revealed to him the significant link between emotional conflicts and physical health conditions.

In examining his own condition, Dr. Hamer realized that his illness was not a random occurrence but a meaningful biological adaptation—a survival mechanism designed to help the body endure significant emotional trauma. The loss of his son triggered a biological conflict tied to survival, which manifested physically in his testicular tissues. This insight laid the foundation for what we now understand about the connection between emotional trauma and physical health.

Similarly, in cases of fibromyalgia, spontaneous remission can be seen through GNM as a natural outcome when underlying emotional conflicts are resolved. Chronic pain, fatigue, and muscle tension—key symptoms of fibromyalgia—often stem from deeply held emotional stresses, such as feelings of inadequacy, prolonged mental strain, or unresolved relational challenges. When these conflicts are recognized and processed, the body no longer needs to sustain the biological adaptation, allowing it to transition into a natural healing phase and leading to what may seem like an "unexpected" recovery.

Understanding Spontaneous Remission in Fibromyalgia

Just as Dr. Hamer understood that his cancer was a response to a significant emotional conflict, individuals with fibromyalgia may find that their path to healing involves addressing similar underlying emotional stresses. Conflicts related to self-worth, relational challenges, or overburdening oneself can initiate biological programs that manifest as the chronic pain and fatigue seen in fibromyalgia. According to GNM, these physical symptoms serve as the body's adaptation to these unresolved emotional stresses.

When these emotional conflicts are resolved, the body no longer has a reason to maintain the biological adaptations, allowing it to move into the healing phase. What once seemed like a miraculous or mysterious recovery can now be recognized as the body's intelligent response to emotional resolution. Through the combined power of belief, emotional healing, and resolution of conflict, spontaneous remission becomes possible, grounded in the body's inherent ability to restore balance and health.

In this view, spontaneous remission is not an anomaly, but rather a testament to the body's potential to heal itself when emotional conflicts are acknowledged and resolved, offering hope for a natural pathway to recovery from fibromyalgia.

The Six Human Needs by Tony Robbins: An Adaptation for Chronic Conditions

At the heart of every decision, action, and emotion lies a set of core needs that influence our behaviour in profound and sometimes unconscious ways. These are not mere desires; they are fundamental human needs that shape the way we experience life. Tony Robbins, a leading authority in personal development, identified these as the Six Human Needs. In the context of chronic conditions like fibromyalgia and chronic fatigue syndrome, understanding these needs is crucial, as these needs can both drive behaviors that exacerbate symptoms and support healing.

Why Understanding the Six Human Needs Matters

Imagine trying to live without food, water, or air. Just as these are essential for physical survival, the Six Human Needs are essential for emotional and psychological well-being. Every action we take attempts to meet one or more of these needs. Unmet needs can contribute to emotional strain, adding to the burden on an already taxed body. Recognizing how these needs impact our lives and learning how to meet them in healthy ways can be transformative, particularly in managing chronic conditions.

For instance, unmet needs for significance or connection might lead a person to behaviors that ultimately increase stress or isolation, perpetuating pain or fatigue. The more aware we become of our needs, the better we can meet them in ways that support our well-being.

The Six Human Needs Explained

Certainty: The Need for Stability and Control

Certainty represents our need for stability, comfort, and predictability. For those with chronic conditions, this often translates into routines, boundaries, and consistency that help stabilize emotions and health amid unpredictable symptoms.

- Positive Vehicles:
    - Practicing saying "no" to demands that exhaust your energy, knowing that setting limits is essential for long-term self-care.

- Establishing supportive routines that honour your body's needs, like rest, gentle exercise, and nourishing meals.
- Building open communication with loved ones to create understanding around your limitations, making room for both empathy and boundaries.

- Example in Practice:
    - Many people with chronic conditions feel pressure to continue supporting family or friends, even to the point of sacrificing their own well-being. Saying "no" to these demands can feel uncomfortable at first due to feelings of guilt or responsibility. However, with time, setting boundaries enables the other person to grow independently while protecting your health. Although it may be challenging initially, this boundary-setting is a positive vehicle for well-being, enabling both personal and relational resilience.
- Negative Vehicles:
    - Sacrificing personal needs to please others, leading to burnout or symptom flare-ups.
    - People-pleasing behaviors that temporarily ease guilt but ultimately undermine well-being.
    - Using avoidance or self-sacrifice to cope, providing short-term relief but reinforcing exhaustion and dependency.

Variety: The Need for Challenge and Change

Variety represents our need for stimulation, change, and novelty. Without it, life feels monotonous and uninspiring. For those managing chronic symptoms, finding balance between stability and variety is key.

- Positive Vehicles:
    - Exploring new hobbies or creative outlets that bring enjoyment without overtaxing physical limits, such as painting, knitting, or learning a new language.

- Engaging in light, spontaneous social activities that bring joy without causing stress.
- Adjusting routines periodically to prevent monotony while maintaining supportive habits.

- Negative Vehicles:
  - Seeking drama or unnecessary conflict as a way to feel engaged.
  - Relying on substances or excessive screen time to escape routine, creating dependency without genuine fulfillment.

Significance: The Need to Feel Important

The need for significance drives us to feel unique and valued. Chronic conditions can challenge this need, often leading to feelings of inadequacy or self-doubt.

- Positive Vehicles:
  - Setting personal goals within your capacity, like learning a new skill or completing small projects that bring a sense of accomplishment.
  - Contributing to supportive communities, such as chronic illness forums, by sharing your journey and encouraging others.
  - Cultivating a sense of self-worth independent of physical health, recognizing your inherent value and contributions.
- Negative Vehicles:
  - Putting others down or engaging in judgmental behaviour to feel superior.
  - Engaging in extreme behaviour or overextending yourself to gain approval.
  - Using self-criticism as a way to draw attention or as a subconscious response to unmet needs.

Love and Connection: The Need for Emotional Bonds

Love and connection are essential to our emotional health. For those with chronic conditions, fostering healthy relationships is vital for both emotional and physical resilience.

- Positive Vehicles:
    - Cultivating meaningful connections through open, honest communication with friends and family.
    - Setting boundaries that protect your health without compromising connection, like scheduling quality time with loved ones that respects your limits.
    - Practicing self-compassion to foster a healthy relationship with yourself, which in turn supports healthier external relationships.
- Negative Vehicles:
    - Becoming overly dependent on others for validation or self-worth.
    - Using physical intimacy as a replacement for emotional closeness, risking imbalance in relationships.
    - Engaging in people-pleasing to avoid rejection, ultimately creating inner stress and resentment.

Growth: The Need for Personal Development

Growth drives us to learn, adapt, and evolve. Chronic conditions can sometimes feel like they inhibit growth, but they also offer unique opportunities for deep personal development.

- Positive Vehicles:
    - Setting achievable goals, like learning mindfulness or relaxation techniques to manage stress.
    - Pursuing knowledge about your condition and self-care strategies, empowering yourself to manage symptoms more effectively.

    - Engaging in self-reflection practices, like journaling or meditation, to build resilience and self-awareness.
- Negative Vehicles:
    - Becoming consumed by self-improvement to the point of burnout or neglecting other needs.
    - Comparing yourself to others or past versions of yourself, leading to frustration or feelings of inadequacy.

Contribution: The Need to Give Beyond Ourselves

Contribution is the need to give to others, to feel that our lives matter beyond ourselves. In the context of chronic illness, this can be met by sharing experiences, supporting others, and finding meaningful ways to give back.

- Positive Vehicles:
    - Volunteering within your capacity, such as mentoring or supporting others with similar challenges.
    - Sharing knowledge or strategies with people navigating similar journeys, fostering a supportive community.
    - Engaging in activities aligned with your values, creating purpose while respecting physical boundaries.
- Negative Vehicles:
    - Overextending yourself to feel valued, risking fatigue or burnout.
    - Contributing for external validation rather than genuine desire to help, leading to potential resentment.

Understanding the Vehicles We Use

In the pursuit of fulfilling these needs, our choices—our "vehicles"—vary widely in quality and impact. Each action we take can be classified by how well it serves us and those around us, with an eye toward balancing the Six Human Needs in ways that support both immediate and long-term well-being.

The Four Classes of Vehicles for Meeting Your Needs

4 classes of vehicles

	Feels Good	Is Good for you	Serves Others	Serves the greater good
Class 1	✓	✓	✓	✓
Class 2	✗	✓	✓	✓
Class 3	✓	✗	✗	✗
Class 4	✗	✗	✗	✗

When it comes to meeting our needs, the methods we choose—referred to here as "vehicles"—can vary widely in their effectiveness and impact. Here's a breakdown of these vehicles into four classes, based on how they impact ourselves and others:

Class 1: The Ideal Vehicles

- Positive Examples: Setting boundaries, practicing mindfulness, and engaging in hobbies that bring both joy and stability.
- Negative Examples: Overextending yourself for validation, people-pleasing at the expense of self-care.

Class 2: The Disciplined Vehicles

- Positive Examples: Saying "no" when necessary to protect your health, developing consistent routines.
- Example in Practice: Many individuals struggle to say "no" to family members who rely heavily on their support. Though challenging at first due to guilt or fear of disappointing others, this disciplined action fosters long-term independence and healthier relationships.

Class 3: The Instant Gratification Vehicles

- Positive Examples: Engaging in light entertainment or social activities as a form of healthy balance.

- Negative Examples: Comfort eating or excessive screen time to escape discomfort, leading to dependency and fatigue.

Class 4: The Destructive Vehicles

- Positive Examples: Practicing humour to deflect negativity, taking short breaks to manage overwhelm.
- Negative Examples: Substance abuse, gossip, or self-sabotaging behaviors that erode trust, well-being, or relationships.

Certainty: The Need for Stability and Control
At a fundamental level, everyone needs certainty—the desire for stability, comfort, and predictability. Certainty provides a sense of safety and control in a world that can often feel chaotic. For those dealing with chronic conditions like fibromyalgia, the need for certainty is especially critical, as the unpredictability of symptoms can lead to feelings of anxiety and vulnerability.

- **In the context of fibromyalgia:**
    - A person may feel out of control due to the unpredictability of their pain, fatigue, or flare-ups, which can heighten anxiety and stress. The need for stability can lead to an increased focus on routines and protective behaviors, such as avoiding certain social events or activities to minimize stress.
    - Additionally, the struggle to control physical symptoms can create an emotional conflict, where individuals may feel trapped in their condition, unable to break free from the limitations it imposes on their life.
- **Response to unmet certainty needs:**
    - When the need for certainty isn't met, individuals might cope by withdrawing from others or over-controlling aspects of their environment. However, this can reinforce feelings of isolation or helplessness, deepening the emotional conflict.

Variety: The Need for Challenge and Change
While certainty is essential, we also have a need for variety—the desire for change, excitement, and new experiences. For those managing chronic conditions, balancing stability with variety can be challenging, as too much unpredictability can worsen symptoms.

- **In the context of fibromyalgia:**
    - Individuals may feel a tension between craving stimulation and fearing the physical toll that new activities might take. A person with fibromyalgia may long for excitement and change but feel trapped in a repetitive routine that limits variety, leading to boredom or restlessness.

    - The desire for variety might manifest in the form of emotional stress or frustration, as individuals seek ways to bring novelty into their lives without compromising their health.

- **Response to unmet variety needs:**
    - When this need for variety isn't met in healthy ways, some may turn to escapism, like excessive screen time or engaging in social drama to add excitement. However, these behaviors can add to emotional stress, ultimately exacerbating symptoms.

Significance: The Need to Feel Important

The need for significance is a powerful driver, reflecting our desire to feel valued and unique. Chronic conditions can challenge this need, as individuals may feel that their identity and contributions are overshadowed by their health challenges.

- **In the context of fibromyalgia:**
    - Many people with fibromyalgia experience feelings of inadequacy or loss of identity, especially if their ability to work, socialize, or engage in meaningful activities is impacted. This can lead to an internal conflict where they feel insignificant or unseen, fuelling frustration and self-doubt.
    - Additionally, societal attitudes toward "invisible" conditions may leave people feeling misunderstood or judged, creating further emotional tension and the need to assert their worth and capabilities.

- **Response to unmet significance needs:**
    - To compensate, individuals might seek validation through external means, such as constantly pushing their limits to prove themselves, sometimes at the cost of worsening symptoms. This drive for significance can lead to cycles of burnout as they attempt to meet this need in unsustainable ways.

Love and Connection: The Need for Emotional Bonds

The need for love and connection is fundamental to well-being. Chronic conditions can create feelings of isolation, either due to physical limitations or due to others' inability to fully understand the struggles involved.

- **In the context of fibromyalgia:**
    - Individuals may feel a "separation conflict," where they experience emotional disconnect or even rejection from friends, family, or colleagues who don't understand their symptoms. Feelings of being a burden or misunderstood can lead to isolation and loneliness.
    - Many find it difficult to set boundaries with loved ones, especially if they feel guilty about needing help or declining invitations. This internal struggle often heightens emotional stress and, in turn, can worsen physical symptoms.
- **Response to unmet connection needs:**
    - When the need for connection goes unmet, people might suppress their emotions, withdraw from loved ones, or overextend themselves to please others. Setting boundaries—even though it may feel difficult initially—is essential for both parties to foster healthy interdependence and prevent emotional burnout.

Growth: The Need for Personal Development
Growth represents the need to learn, expand, and evolve. Chronic conditions can make personal development feel challenging, especially if there is a sense of being "stuck" in a cycle of pain or fatigue.

- **In the context of fibromyalgia:**
    - The journey of managing a chronic condition can feel limiting, as individuals may fear that they won't be able to pursue personal goals or reach their potential. When personal growth is hindered by the condition, it can lead to feelings of frustration or stagnation.
    - Growth, however, can also manifest through self-compassion, resilience, and adaptability, which can provide valuable lessons in navigating life's challenges.
- **Response to unmet growth needs:**

- Avoiding growth entirely due to fear of worsening symptoms can lead to emotional stagnation. Conversely, setting small, achievable goals, such as learning coping techniques or developing creative hobbies, can provide a sense of accomplishment and fulfillment that supports both mental and physical well-being.

Contribution: The Need to Give Beyond Ourselves
Contribution is the need to make a positive impact, feeling that our lives matter beyond ourselves. Chronic conditions can complicate this need, especially if physical limitations impact one's ability to give in conventional ways.

- **In the context of fibromyalgia:**
  - People may feel a loss of purpose if they're unable to contribute in the same ways they once did, such as through work or caregiving. This can lead to feelings of sadness or a diminished sense of self-worth.
  - Exploring new ways to contribute, however, like sharing experiences, supporting others facing similar conditions, or engaging in community projects within one's capacity, can foster a renewed sense of purpose and fulfillment.
- **Response to unmet contribution needs:**
  - When contribution needs are neglected, individuals might experience feelings of emptiness or purposelessness. Finding adaptive ways to give back—whether through advocacy, creativity, or peer support—can fulfil this need in a way that aligns with their health.

The Balance of Needs and Health

When these six needs are met in healthy ways, individuals feel balanced and resilient, even while navigating chronic conditions. However, when these needs are unmet or met in unhealthy ways, they can contribute to emotional conflicts, which German New Medicine suggests may influence physical symptoms. Recognizing and addressing these needs, especially in the context of chronic health challenges, can provide a framework for understanding one's behaviors and emotions, supporting both mental and physical resilience.

Transition: Uncovering the Character Within

As we delve deeper into understanding the Six Human Needs, it becomes clear that each of us has unique ways of meeting these needs, whether positively or negatively. But there's something intriguing and profound when we consider this in relation to ourselves—who is it, within us, that drives us to meet our needs in ways that don't always serve us well?

Who is this Character Within You?

Have you ever noticed a part of you that seems to act on its own, making choices you know aren't in your best interest? Perhaps it's the part that chooses to overindulge in food, even though you've promised yourself you'd eat healthier. Or maybe it's the part that avoids important tasks, choosing procrastination and distraction over productivity. You know these actions aren't beneficial, yet somehow, you find yourself repeating them. Who is this character that seems to steer your ship off course?

We all have these parts within us—characters that take over when we're stressed, tired, or overwhelmed. They show up when our needs are not being met and seem to offer a quick fix, a temporary relief, or a way to escape.

Reflect on Your Own Character

Think for a moment: What do you call this part of you? Is it "The Critic," who harshly judges you and others to feel significant? Or maybe it's "The Escapist," who reaches for distractions, like mindless scrolling or binge-watching, to avoid uncomfortable feelings? Perhaps it's "The Pleaser," who sacrifices personal needs to gain love and connection, but ends up feeling empty and resentful.

This character has been with you for a long time, playing a role in how you've learned to survive and navigate the world. But is this character truly serving you? Or is it holding you back from living authentically and healthily?

The Shadow Self: An Adaptive Protector

This character within you is not a stranger but a part of you—your shadow self. It's an adaptive mechanism that formed in response to past pain, unmet needs, and emotional conflicts. While it may have protected you once, it can become a hindrance when it takes over your decisions and actions.

The shadow self often emerges when we are trying to meet our needs in ways that are not aligned with our true selves. For example, a man who feels emasculated might develop a shadow character who becomes overly dominant or controlling to compensate for feelings of inadequacy. Or someone who feels unworthy of love might create a character who constantly seeks validation from others, leading to a cycle of dependency and disappointment.

Questioning the Shadow: Who is Really in Control?

Ask yourself: "When does this character show up most in my life? How does it make me feel afterward? What are the long-term consequences of letting this character run the show?"

By becoming aware of this shadow character, you gain the power to make conscious choices. You can begin to shift from reacting unconsciously to life's challenges to responding with awareness and intention.

Introducing the Shadow Archetypes

In the following section, we will explore the concept of shadow archetypes—different forms that this character can take, depending on our unique experiences and emotional conflicts. Understanding these archetypes helps us see the role they play in our lives and how they impact our health and well-being.

By recognizing these characters and their influence, we can start the journey of integrating them, transforming them from saboteurs to allies. This is the first step in reclaiming your true self, free from the unconscious patterns that have held you back.

Understanding the Four Shadow Archetypes:

Recognizing Common Behaviors and Relationship Dynamics

Everyone has shadow aspects within them—parts of themselves that have fractured away as a form of protection. These shadows are not inherently negative; they develop as adaptive mechanisms, shaped by early life experiences, societal pressures, or emotional trauma. They act as protectors when expressing our true self might feel unsafe or unacceptable. Over time, these adaptive parts become our default ways of coping with difficult people, challenging circumstances, or emotional pain.

The shadow self exists in contrast to the true self—the part of us that is authentic, open, and aligned with our core identity. The true self is often suppressed because it feels vulnerable in a world that demands conformity, approval, or survival. In its place, the shadow steps forward, using behaviors and strategies that help us navigate difficult situations, but which may not always serve our long-term well-being.

These shadow behaviors can seem harmful or counterproductive on the surface, but they've developed for a reason. Understanding them with compassion allows us to see how they've protected us in various contexts. In this section, we'll explore four common shadow archetypes—the Blamer, Placator, Computer, and Distractor—and look at how they shape our relationships and life choices.

The Purpose of the Shadow

The shadow doesn't form randomly; it is context-dependent, circumstance-dependent, and people-dependent. Different aspects of the shadow may arise in different situations or with different people. For example, someone may adopt the Placator role in relationships to avoid conflict, while embodying the computer role at work to suppress emotions and maintain control.

These shadow behaviors are adaptive responses to a world where being our true selves may not always feel safe. While they serve as protection, they can also lead to patterns that hinder personal growth and even contribute to physical health issues when left unchecked. By understanding the shadow and how it operates, we can begin to recognize when and why we suppress our true self and make more conscious choices.

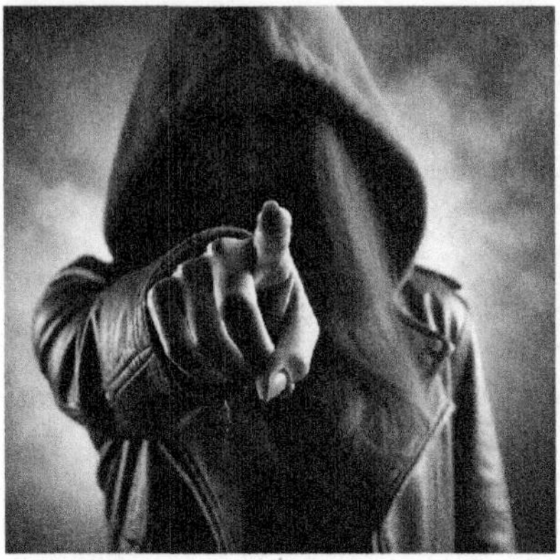 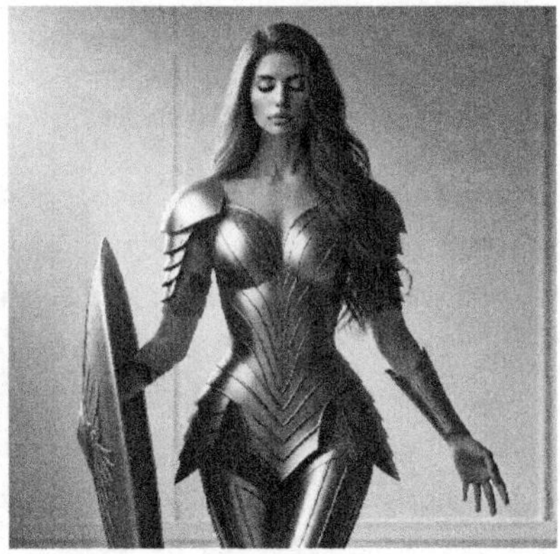

1. The Blamer

The **Blamer** is a shadow archetype that deflects responsibility and seeks to place fault on others as a way to protect the self from feelings of inadequacy or guilt. Initially, the Blamer points outward, accusing others of causing the circumstances and results in their life. However, when this outward blame fails to provide the desired outcome, the Blamer often turns the blame inwards, leading to deep feelings of self-criticism and guilt. This paradox mirrors the behaviour of the **Placator**, whose initial response is to blame inwardly, but when that no longer serves them, they too project blame outwardly.

Origins in Family Dynamics

The Blamer often develops in environments where individuals felt powerless or unheard as children. If a child grows up in a home where their voice or needs were not validated, they may learn to deflect responsibility or blame others as a defence mechanism. This behaviour is often rooted in a deeper fear of inadequacy or rejection.

- **Family Dynamics**: In families where one parent was overly critical or distant, a child may feel constant pressure to be "good enough." If they didn't receive the validation they needed, they may have turned to blaming others as a way to protect themselves from feeling vulnerable or insignificant.
- **Tony Robbins' Question**: "Whose love did you crave most—your mother's or your father's?" In many cases, the Blamer craved the love of a distant or overly critical parent and learned that by shifting blame or deflecting responsibility, they could avoid emotional pain or criticism.

- **Emotional Protection**: The Blamer's need to deflect responsibility often arises from an internal sense of inadequacy, where outward blame becomes a shield against feelings of guilt, failure, or not being enough.

Common Behaviors of the Blamer:

- **Backbiting**: Speaking negatively about others behind their backs, often to deflect attention from one's own shortcomings.
- **Negative Self-Talk**: Initially deflecting outward, but eventually blaming oneself, thinking, "I'm not good enough," or "It's all my fault."
- **Seeing the Negative**: Focusing on the flaws in others, but eventually noticing only the flaws within oneself.
- **Gaslighting**: Manipulating others into questioning their reality to avoid taking responsibility, and later questioning their own reality when the blame turns inward.
- **Substance Use as an Escape**: Turning to substances like alcohol or cigarettes to escape both self-blame and the discomfort of blaming others.
- **Sex and Pornography as an Escape**: Using compulsive sexual behaviour or pornography to numb feelings of inadequacy and avoid both inward and outward blame.
- **Controlling and Bullying**: Using intimidation to dominate others and avoid facing one's own shortcomings, but eventually blaming oneself for the lack of control.

Relationship Dynamics:

The **Blamer** often attracts partners who are submissive or who have a strong need to please. This dynamic allows the Blamer to dominate, but eventually, the imbalance creates resentment and stagnation for both individuals. Similarly, the Placator attracts more dominant partners but may also flip the blame outward when their strategy of self-blame doesn't work.

Transitioning from Blamer to Warrior

The empowered version of the Blamer is the **Warrior**. Where the Blamer deflects responsibility to protect themselves from feelings of inadequacy, the Warrior faces challenges head-on with courage and strength. The Warrior doesn't blame others or themselves; instead, they take responsibility for their actions and decisions, understanding that personal empowerment lies in owning their circumstances rather than deflecting or internalizing blame.

The **Warrior** embodies a powerful balance of **feminine and masculine energy**. While the **masculine energy** of the Warrior is seen in their ability to take action, assert control, and move forward, the **feminine energy** brings emotional vulnerability and openness. The Warrior knows that true strength lies in being both courageous and vulnerable—allowing space for their emotions while taking full ownership of their role in creating change.

Feminine Energy and Vulnerability in the Warrior

For those who identify strongly with the **Blamer**, transitioning to the Warrior requires embracing both your natural sense of strength and your vulnerability. Vulnerability is not a weakness, but rather a powerful tool that the Warrior uses to connect with themselves and others. By allowing themselves to be open and emotionally authentic, the Warrior is able to form stronger relationships and navigate challenges without feeling the need to deflect blame.

- **Owning Your Power**: The Warrior knows that pointing fingers at others or criticizing oneself is an avoidance of true power. Ask yourself, "What would happen if I took full responsibility for my actions, without blame?"
- **Embracing Vulnerability**: The Warrior understands that vulnerability doesn't diminish their strength—it enhances it. How can you allow yourself to be open and emotionally honest without falling into blame or self-criticism?

Reflection and Exercise:

Take a moment to reflect on how the **Blamer** shows up in your life. The goal is to explore these patterns without judgment, with empathy and self-compassion.

Questions for Reflection:

- Which of these behaviors do you recognize in yourself?
- List any behaviors that resonate with you. It might be outward blame toward others or inward self-criticism. Which pattern feels more familiar to you?
- Do you notice a shift from outward blame to self-blame when your initial strategy doesn't work?
- Think about a time when blaming others didn't solve the issue. Did you then turn the blame inward, criticizing yourself for the situation?
- In your relationships, do you notice dynamics where blame cycles between others and yourself?
- Reflect on any patterns in your relationships where the blame starts outward and then moves inward, or vice versa. How does this affect your emotional well-being and connection with others?

Writing Exercise:

On a sheet of paper, write down the behaviors and relationship dynamics you recognize from the **Blamer**. Acknowledge both the outward blame you may have directed at others and the inward blame you've turned on yourself. As you write, practice self-compassion—this exercise is not about judgment but about understanding your shadow patterns.

Ask yourself, **How has this pattern served me in the past?** Sit with that question and acknowledge how both blaming outwardly and inwardly may have been a way to protect yourself. Remember, as you reflect, self-empathy and self-compassion are key to understanding your shadow. Simply acknowledging these patterns without judgment is the first step toward healing.

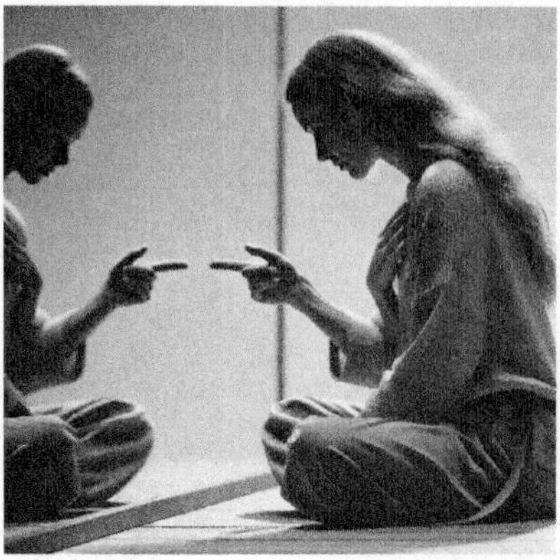 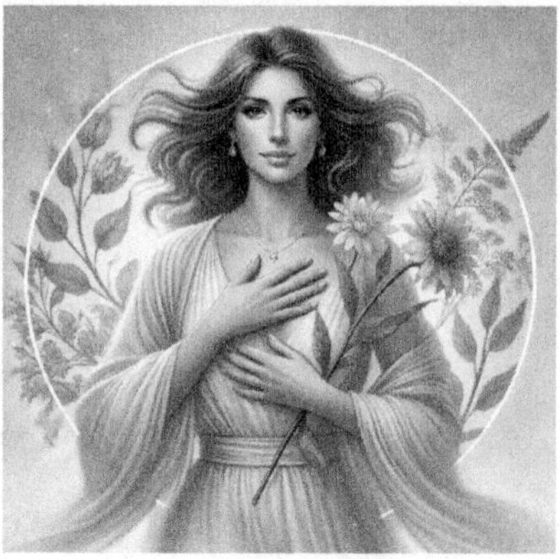

2. The Placator

The **Placator** is a shadow that seeks to avoid conflict and gain approval by excessively pleasing others, often at the expense of their own needs and authenticity. Initially, the Placator tends to blame themselves for problems, bending over backward to appease others. However, when this strategy fails to meet their needs or resolve the issue, they may project their frustrations outward, blaming others. This is the inverse of the **Blamer**, who begins by blaming others and then turns inward when their strategy doesn't work.

Origins in Family Dynamics

The Placator usually forms in households where peacekeeping or appeasement was necessary to maintain harmony. As children, they may have learned to prioritize the needs and emotions of others to avoid conflict or gain approval. This shadow is rooted in the fear of rejection or abandonment.

- **Family Dynamics**: Placators often come from homes where one or both parents were emotionally volatile or difficult to please. The child learned that in order to maintain harmony or avoid conflict, they had to sacrifice their own needs and become the "pleaser."
- **Tony Robbins' Question**: "Who did you have to be for that person?" Placators often find that they had to be the "good child" or the peacekeeper in their family, avoiding their own needs in favour of maintaining the love or attention of a caregiver.
- **Emotional Protection**: This shadow develops as a way to protect the individual from conflict or disapproval. By constantly putting others first, the Placator avoids the emotional turmoil that comes with being true to their own desires or needs.

Common Behaviors of the Placator:

- **Not Being True to Yourself**: Engaging in conversations or actions that don't align with your true feelings to avoid conflict.
- **Self-Sacrifice**: Prioritizing others' needs over your own, even when it leads to emotional or physical exhaustion.
- **Over-Apologizing**: Frequently apologizing, even when there's no need, often as a way to avoid conflict or disapproval.
- **Seeking External Validation**: Relying heavily on others' approval to feel good about yourself, often at the cost of your self-worth.
- **Using Food or Shopping for Comfort**: Overeating or engaging in impulsive shopping as a way to soothe emotional distress when internal blame becomes too overwhelming.
- **Social Media Addiction**: Constantly seeking validation through likes, comments, or attention on social media platforms to fill the void created by self-blame.
- **Overly Submissive and Manipulative**: Allowing others to dominate or manipulate you, while subtly manipulating situations to maintain approval and avoid confrontation.

Relationship Dynamics:

The **Placator** often attracts dominant or controlling partners, leading to an unhealthy relationship dynamic where the Placator's needs are consistently overlooked. This can result in emotional burnout, as the Placator gives and gives without receiving. Like the **Blamer**, the Placator can shift from self-blame to blaming others when their strategy of pleasing no longer works.

Transitioning from Placator to Lover

The empowered version of the **Placator** is the **Lover**. The **Lover** understands that true connection and love come from a place of **authenticity** and **emotional balance** rather than seeking approval at the cost of their own needs. The **Lover** nurtures relationships, not by self-sacrifice, but through mutual care, honesty, and self-worth.

Where the **Placator** may compromise their own needs to keep others happy, the **Lover** expresses both **feminine vulnerability** and **strength** with balance. The **feminine energy** of the Lover is soft, empathetic, and nurturing, yet it is also grounded in self-respect and assertiveness. The **Lover** knows that love begins with self-love, and only by honouring one's own needs can true connection with others flourish.

Feminine Energy and Vulnerability in the Lover

Transitioning from the **Placator** to the **Lover** requires embracing both emotional vulnerability and personal boundaries. The **Lover** understands that vulnerability isn't about losing yourself in others, but about showing your true self without fear of rejection.

- **Embrace Self-Worth**: The Lover knows that love starts within. Ask yourself, "How can I honour my own needs while still showing care for others?"
- **Balance Giving with Receiving**: The **Lover** maintains balance by giving and receiving in relationships. Reflect on whether your relationships allow for mutual care or if they are one-sided.

Reflection and Exercise:

Take a moment to reflect on how the **Placator** might resonate with you. This is a time for introspection and compassion—exploring these patterns without judgment can lead to greater self-awareness.

Questions for Reflection:

- Do you recognize any of these behaviors in yourself?
- Take a moment to list any of the behaviors above that feel familiar. Have you found yourself apologizing too much, or sacrificing your needs to keep the peace? Write down what resonates most.
- Do you tend to blame yourself when things go wrong in your relationships or work?
- Think about how often you internalize blame when things don't go as planned. Do you feel the need to fix situations by overextending yourself, even if it's not your fault?

- When your self-blame doesn't work, do you eventually turn your frustration outward?
- Reflect on whether you've ever shifted from self-blame to blaming others after realizing that constantly pleasing people doesn't resolve the deeper issues. How has this shift impacted your relationships?

Writing Exercise:

Using a journal or notebook, list the behaviors and relationship dynamics you identify with as a **Placator**. Acknowledge how often you've blamed yourself for problems, and how you may have sought approval by sacrificing your needs.

Next, reflect on whether your strategy of self-blame and placating others has ever shifted into outward frustration or blame. What patterns emerge when you're no longer able to maintain the peace through self-sacrifice?

As you write, remember to approach this exercise with self-compassion. You're not judging yourself, but rather acknowledging the shadow behaviors that have played a role in your life. Understanding these behaviors is the first step toward freeing yourself from the **Placator's** grip.

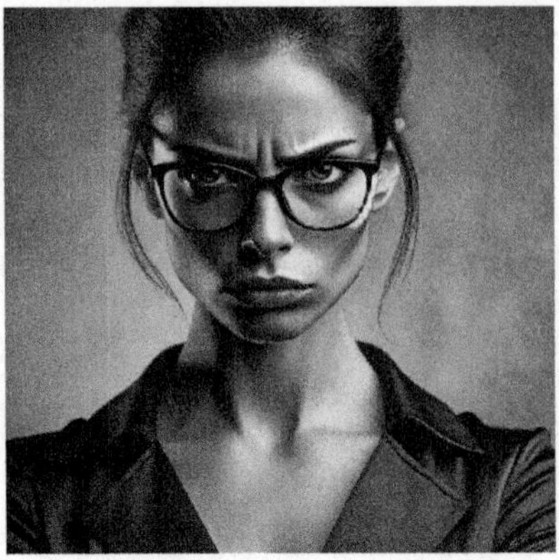 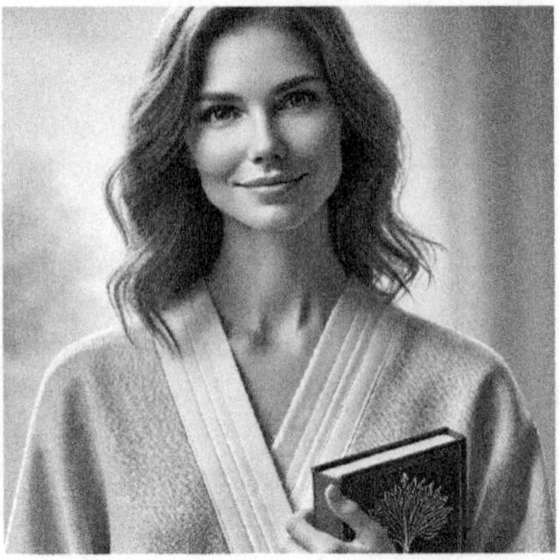

3. The Computer

The **Computer** is a shadow that suppresses emotions, relying heavily on logic and intellect to navigate life, often at the cost of emotional connection and empathy. This shadow tends to overanalyse situations, avoiding vulnerability and keeping emotions at arm's length. The **Computer** sees emotional expression as a weakness and will often rationalize away feelings rather than confronting them head-on.

Origins in Family Dynamics

The Computer often emerges from environments where emotions were undervalued or ignored. If a child grew up in a family where intellectual achievement or rational behaviour was prioritized over emotional connection, they may learn to suppress their feelings and rely on logic to navigate life.

- **Family Dynamics**: Computers often come from homes where emotions were dismissed or seen as a weakness. Perhaps a parent was emotionally unavailable or overly focused on academic or career success, leaving the child feeling that emotions were irrelevant or distracting.
- **Tony Robbins' Question**: "Whose love did you crave most, and how did you have to behave to get it?" Computers may have learned that in order to gain the approval of a parent, they needed to be rational, in control, and unemotional. Vulnerability would have been seen as a weakness.
- **Emotional Protection**: The Computer uses logic as a defence against emotional vulnerability. By focusing on intellect and control,

they protect themselves from feeling exposed or weak in the emotional realm.

Common Behaviors of the Computer:

- **Emotional Detachment**: Avoiding deep emotional connections by staying focused on facts and logic.
- **Over-Analysing**: Constantly analysing situations to avoid dealing with underlying emotions.
- **Rationalizing Away Emotions**: Justifying emotional experiences with logic, rather than acknowledging and feeling them.
- **Avoiding Vulnerability**: Refusing to show or acknowledge vulnerability, even when it's necessary for deeper connection.
- **Using Substances to Stay "In Control"**: Using stimulants like caffeine or energy drinks to maintain focus and avoid emotional experiences.
- **Addiction to Work or Intellectual Pursuits**: Using work or intellectual achievements as a distraction from emotional issues, prioritizing productivity over emotional well-being.

Relationship Dynamics:

The **Computer** often attracts emotionally expressive or volatile partners, leading to emotional disconnection and a lack of depth in relationships. This dynamic may reinforce the **Computer's** tendency to avoid emotions, creating a cycle where they further withdraw into logic and reason, avoiding the emotional chaos of their partner.

Transitioning from Computer to Guru

The empowered version of the **Computer** is the **Guru**. Where the **Computer** avoids emotions and clings to intellect, the **Guru** integrates both logic and emotion to create deep wisdom. The **Guru** understands that true clarity comes from embracing both the intellect and the heart, using their deep knowledge to guide others with compassion and emotional insight.

The **Guru** embodies a powerful balance of **masculine logic** and **feminine emotional intelligence**. Where the **Computer** sees vulnerability as a weakness, the **Guru** views it as a strength—knowing that vulnerability allows for deeper connection and greater emotional freedom.

Feminine Energy and Vulnerability in the Guru

Transitioning from the **Computer** to the **Guru** requires embracing emotional vulnerability and developing empathy. The **Guru** knows that emotions are not something to be controlled or avoided but to be felt and integrated alongside intellectual understanding.

- **Embrace Emotional Intelligence**: The **Guru** knows that emotions are valuable sources of wisdom. Ask yourself, "How can I honour my emotions without losing my logical perspective?"
- **Balance Logic with Compassion**: The **Guru** holds both logic and compassion equally. How can you bring more emotional presence into your relationships and still maintain your sense of reason?

Reflection and Exercise:

If you relate to the **Computer**, it's important to approach this reflection with self-compassion. The goal is to explore how logic and emotional detachment serve you and, perhaps, where they limit your emotional connections.

Questions for Reflection:

- **Which of these behaviors do you recognize in yourself?** Write down any behaviors that resonate with you. Do you notice yourself relying on logic and analysis to navigate difficult situations, while avoiding emotional expression?
- **Do you tend to rationalize your emotions or push them aside?** Think of moments where you've justified your emotions or simply brushed them away. How often do you choose to stay "in control" rather than allow yourself to feel vulnerable?
- **In your relationships, do you find yourself withdrawing emotionally or overanalysing interactions?** Reflect on whether you tend to disengage from emotionally charged conversations or use intellect to distance yourself. How does this impact the emotional depth of your relationships?

Writing Exercise:

Using a notebook, write down how often you prioritize logic and intellectual pursuits over emotional expression. Do you notice patterns of emotional avoidance? Acknowledge these behaviors without judgment.

Next, ask yourself: **What would it feel like to express your emotions more openly?** Reflect on times when emotional vulnerability felt risky and how you navigated that. The goal isn't to change immediately but to become more aware of when and why you avoid emotional connection.

Remember: As with any shadow, the **Computer's** role is to protect you. By acknowledging these patterns, you can bring more balance into your life—honouring both logic and emotion as essential parts of your well-being.

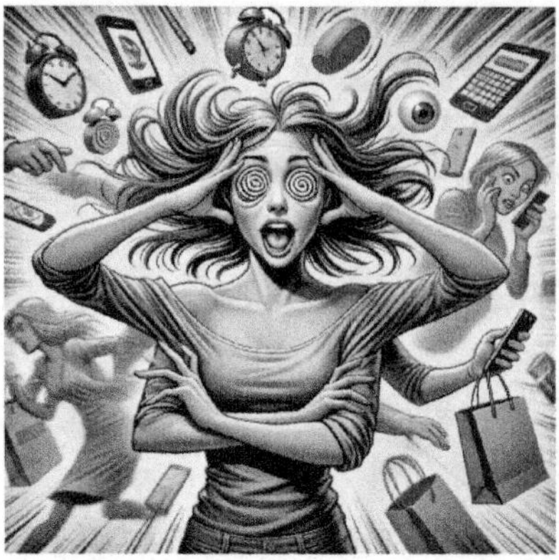 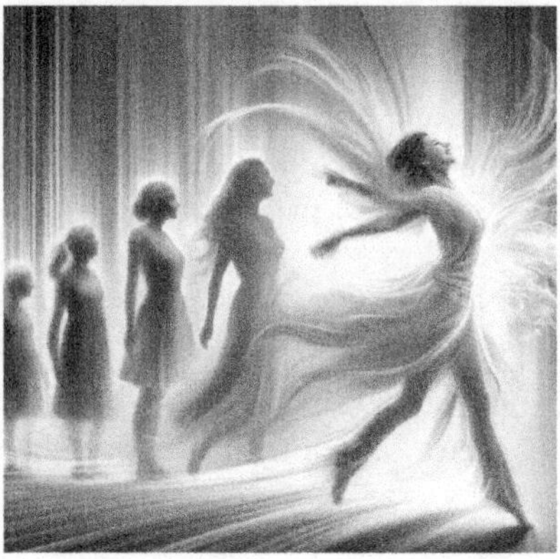

4. The Distractor

The **Distractor** is a shadow that uses humour, avoidance, or distractions to evade deeper issues or emotions. Instead of facing difficult conversations or feelings, the **Distractor** diverts attention through procrastination, sarcasm, or compulsive behaviors. While this strategy helps them temporarily escape discomfort, it often prevents deeper emotional growth.

Origins in Family Dynamics

The Distractor often develops in environments where emotions or conflicts were overwhelming or too intense to confront. Instead of facing these situations, the Distractor learns to divert attention away from uncomfortable emotions or difficult conversations, often through humour, avoidance, or procrastination.

- **Family Dynamics**: Distractors may come from chaotic homes where conflict or emotional expression was overwhelming. In some cases, they may have been raised in environments where their emotional needs were not met, causing them to learn that distraction was the safest way to cope.
- **Tony Robbins' Question**: "Who did you have to be to maintain peace?" Distractors may have been the "funny one" or the one who avoided serious discussions in order to maintain peace in the household. They learned to avoid emotional depth as a way to protect themselves from conflict or emotional overwhelm.
- **Emotional Protection**: The Distractor uses humour or avoidance to evade deeper emotional pain or unresolved conflicts. Distraction

becomes a tool for staying safe and not confronting uncomfortable realities, but at the cost of emotional depth.

Common Behaviors of the Distractor:

- **Avoiding Difficult Conversations**: Steering conversations away from serious or uncomfortable topics, using humour or distraction to avoid engagement.
- **Procrastination**: Delaying tasks, particularly those that require confronting difficult emotions or situations.
- **Substance Use as a Distraction**: Turning to alcohol, recreational drugs, or entertainment to numb feelings or avoid personal issues.
- **Compulsive Consumption**: Engaging in binge-watching, social media scrolling, or compulsive shopping to escape emotional pain.
- **Overly Sarcastic and Shouting Excessively**: Using sarcasm or shouting to deflect attention from serious issues, keeping things light or chaotic to avoid emotional depth.

Relationship Dynamics:

The **Distractor** may attract chaotic or unpredictable partners, keeping them distracted from their own deeper issues. Alternatively, they may end up with stable partners who grow frustrated over time due to the Distractor's inability to engage in meaningful conversations or emotional depth.

Transitioning from Distractor to Jester

The empowered version of the **Distractor** is the **Jester**. Where the **Distractor** avoids emotional depth through distractions and humour, the **Jester** brings a joyful, light-hearted energy while remaining fully connected to their emotions. The **Jester** can laugh and bring fun into life but does not use humour to avoid vulnerability. Instead, they embrace both playfulness and emotional authenticity, knowing that the two can coexist.

The **Jester** balances **feminine vulnerability** and **masculine playfulness**. They don't shy away from difficult emotions but allow themselves to experience them while still seeing the joy and lightness in life. The **Jester** teaches us that it is possible to face life's challenges with a smile, but not at the cost of avoiding the truth within ourselves.

Feminine Energy and Vulnerability in the Jester

Transitioning from the **Distractor** to the **Jester** involves embracing your **vulnerability** while also maintaining your sense of fun and creativity. The **Jester** knows that it's okay to be vulnerable and emotionally honest, while still being light-hearted and playful.

- **Embrace Playfulness with Depth**: The **Jester** knows that fun doesn't have to mean avoidance. How can you bring playfulness into your life while also remaining connected to your emotions?
- **Allow for Emotional Expression**: The **Jester** expresses emotions openly. Ask yourself, "How can I use humour to connect more deeply, rather than to deflect?"

Reflection and Exercise:

If you relate to the **Distractor**, this reflection is an opportunity to bring awareness to how avoidance or distraction plays a role in your life. The aim is to acknowledge these behaviors without judgment.

Questions for Reflection:

- **Which of these behaviors resonate with you?** Write down any behaviors from the **Distractor** shadow that feel familiar. Have you found yourself using humour, sarcasm, or distractions to avoid important conversations or emotions?
- **Do you procrastinate when faced with tasks that involve emotional depth or discomfort?** Reflect on times when you've delayed dealing with a task or situation because it required confronting emotions or deeper issues. How does procrastination serve as a protective mechanism for you?
- **In your relationships, do you notice a pattern of steering away from serious conversations or relying on distractions?** Consider how your relationships may be affected by your tendency to avoid emotional depth. Do you attract chaotic dynamics to keep yourself distracted, or have you frustrated those who want deeper engagement?

Writing Exercise:

Take some time to journal about how distraction and avoidance have played a role in your life. What emotions or issues have you been evading? List out specific instances when you used humour, substances, or other distractions to avoid dealing with deeper feelings.

As you write, focus on self-compassion. This exercise is not about criticizing yourself but about bringing awareness to patterns that have helped you cope in the past. Once these patterns are acknowledged, you can begin the process of transforming them into more empowering behaviors.

Rediscovering the True Self: The Roots of Our Authentic Identity

In our journey of self-discovery, we must reconnect with the essence of who we were before the world shaped us. The true self—our most authentic identity—is not something we need to create; it's something we need to rediscover.

Reflecting on early childhood helps to uncover traits of the true self that were present before societal expectations and conditioning began to shape our behaviors. Here are key examples of these traits:

Natural Curiosity:

A child is naturally curious, asking endless questions about the world around them—"Why is the sky blue?" or "How do birds fly?" This curiosity is a direct expression of the authentic self, representing an unfiltered interest in the world. It's only later in life that we begin to fear asking "silly" questions, suppressing this natural desire for exploration.

Spontaneous Expression of Emotions:

A toddler may laugh uncontrollably at something they find funny or cry openly when they feel sad or hurt. This raw emotional expression is the true self, unguarded and honest. Over time, we learn to filter and suppress our emotions to conform to societal expectations, but the authentic self always seeks to express feelings freely.

Play and Imagination:

Children often spend hours immersed in imaginative play, creating entire worlds out of a simple cardboard box or pretending to be superheroes. This imaginative freedom is a hallmark of the true self, where creativity flows without the constraints of reality or judgment.

Unconditional Love and Affection:

A child might run up to a parent or sibling and give them a hug without hesitation. This spontaneous show of affection reflects the true self's capacity for love and connection, uninhibited by the fear of rejection or the need for reciprocation.

Honest Responses:

When asked a question, a young child often answers with complete honesty, without concern for social norms or the consequences of their answer. This blunt honesty is a reflection of the true self, which values authenticity over social niceties.

Pursuit of Joy:

Whether it's dancing around the room or splashing in puddles, a child pursues joy for its own sake, without worrying about getting dirty or what others think. This pure enjoyment is a reflection of the true self's desire to seek fulfillment and happiness.

Fearless Exploration:

A child might wander off to explore a new area of the playground without any sense of danger. This fearless curiosity is the true self's drive to experience life fully and uninhibitedly, before learned fears and societal restrictions take over.

Unique Preferences:

A child's preferences—for a certain toy, food, or activity—aren't shaped by what others expect but rather by what resonates deeply with them. These individual preferences showcase the true self's unfiltered likes and dislikes, unshaped by external opinions.

Innate Sense of Justice:

Children often have a strong sense of fairness and will insist that rules are followed or that everyone gets an equal share. This is the true self's natural inclination toward equity and justice, which only later becomes muddled by societal expectations to conform or compromise.

Raw Creativity:

A child may draw the sky purple or name their imaginary friend something completely unique, demonstrating the true self's boundless creativity. This creative freedom is part of the authentic self, unrestrained by the conventions of reality or logic.

Shadows and Chronic Conditions: Connecting Archetypes to Physical Symptoms

Drawing from German New Medicine (GNM), META-Health, and the principles outlined in *The Human Reboot*, we can hypothesize how certain shadow archetypes might contribute to chronic conditions such as fibromyalgia. Chronic conditions like fibromyalgia are often linked to deep emotional conflicts involving themes of self-worth, helplessness, and stress that remains unresolved over time. These emotional struggles can manifest physically as symptoms like widespread pain, fatigue, and sensitivity, characteristic of fibromyalgia. Let's explore how each of the four shadow archetypes might relate to these chronic health challenges.

It's essential to remind ourselves that identifying with a particular shadow archetype or noticing certain behavioural patterns doesn't mean someone will develop a chronic condition like fibromyalgia. As previously discussed in the Six Human Needs section, acting out certain behaviors unproductively doesn't directly lead to physical illness. This understanding helps us become more aware of potential emotional conflicts without implying a deterministic link to disease.

1. **The Blamer**
    - **Potential Chronic Health Impact:** Those with a Blamer archetype might experience fibromyalgia symptoms as they deflect responsibility for their own needs and focus on external sources for their difficulties. This archetype often feels powerless and perceives inadequacy in managing life's demands, which can generate stress that settles into the body as chronic pain and fatigue.
    - **Conflict Theme:** Self-devaluation and inadequacy related to personal worth or feeling unsupported. The Blamer's unresolved feelings of frustration and helplessness may amplify tension in the body, contributing to the persistent pain and sensitivity associated with fibromyalgia.
2. **The Placator**
    - **Potential Chronic Health Impact:** Individuals embodying the Placator archetype frequently sacrifice their needs to please others, which can lead to suppressed feelings of frustration, resentment, or sadness. This constant

suppression contributes to stress that remains unresolved, a factor often linked to fibromyalgia in GNM. The Placator's difficulty in asserting themselves, along with a tendency to avoid conflict, leaves them carrying an emotional burden that can manifest as chronic fatigue and muscle pain.

- **Conflict Theme:** Emotional separation from self and others due to prioritizing others' needs over their own, leading to suppressed anger and frustration. The Placator's avoidance of expressing their true needs can result in physical manifestations of their internal struggle.

3. **The Computer**

   - **Potential Chronic Health Impact:** The Computer archetype often suppresses emotional responses, relying heavily on logic to avoid vulnerability. By dismissing or ignoring emotional needs, they create a disconnect between mind and body, which can lead to an accumulation of stress in the form of chronic tension, fatigue, and fibromyalgia symptoms. Their preference for intellectualizing rather than addressing emotions can contribute to persistent bodily discomfort and fatigue.

   - **Conflict Theme:** Emotional disconnect, as they struggle to acknowledge or express their inner experiences. This emotional restraint can create ongoing tension in the body, contributing to pain and discomfort as the suppressed emotional energy seeks a physical outlet.

4. **The Distractor**

   - **Potential Chronic Health Impact:** The Distractor often avoids emotional discomfort by relying on humour, distractions, or other avoidance tactics, which leaves deep-seated issues unaddressed. For those with fibromyalgia, this evasion can lead to chronic stress, as the emotional weight remains unresolved. The Distractor's reluctance to confront their emotions directly may contribute to ongoing stress that manifests in physical symptoms, such as widespread pain and hypersensitivity.

- **Conflict Theme:** Avoidance of emotional discomfort and unresolved self-worth conflicts. This reluctance to face difficult emotions or conflicts results in an emotional strain that may surface as physical symptoms.

Conclusion: Identifying Shadows and Their Role in Chronic Health Conditions

While each shadow archetype can potentially contribute to chronic health issues, individuals who identify with the Blamer and Placator archetypes may be particularly affected. These archetypes often harbour unresolved conflicts surrounding self-worth, caregiving, and the need to please others, all of which are potential contributors to chronic conditions like fibromyalgia in GNM. Recognizing these shadows provides an opportunity to address underlying conflicts and unresolved emotions, which may lead to improvements in physical health. However, it's important to remember that identifying with a shadow does not mean that one will develop a chronic condition. This understanding is intended to foster awareness and encourage healing through shadow work, emotional integration, and conflict resolution.

Understanding the Roles We Play in Toxic Relationships

Having examined how our shadow selves and unmet needs can influence chronic health conditions, it's important to delve into how these inner conflicts play out in relationships. When we're unaware of our shadows and driven by unfulfilled needs, we may find ourselves repeatedly caught in patterns that contribute to emotional stress. One common and particularly detrimental pattern is represented by the Drama Triangle.

Developed by Dr. Stephen Karpman, the Drama Triangle outlines three roles that people often assume in unhealthy relationship dynamics: the Victim, the Persecutor, and the Rescuer. Each role serves as a way of meeting unmet needs, but often in ways that reinforce negative emotional cycles. Becoming aware of the Drama Triangle helps us recognize how these roles perpetuate conflict and stress, potentially exacerbating underlying emotional conflicts that contribute to conditions like fibromyalgia.

When we habitually adopt one of these roles, we can become trapped in a cycle of tension and stress, which can worsen unresolved conflicts and contribute to physical symptoms, including chronic pain and fatigue. Recognizing these roles and understanding our part in the cycle is the first step toward freeing ourselves from these patterns and meeting our needs in healthier, more constructive ways.

In the following section, we'll explore each role within the Drama Triangle and its connection to unmet needs and shadow behaviors. By becoming aware of these patterns, we can start making conscious choices that support our physical and emotional well-being and contribute to healthier, more fulfilling relationships.

Unravelling the Roles We Play in Toxic Relationships

The Drama Triangle, developed by Dr. Stephen Karpman, provides a powerful framework for understanding the unproductive roles we often assume in relationships: the Victim, the Persecutor, and the Rescuer. While these roles may feel familiar and sometimes even justified, they often create a cycle of stress and unresolved emotional conflict, potentially impacting our physical health and contributing to chronic conditions like fibromyalgia. Understanding these roles can help us identify patterns that may perpetuate emotional and physical stress, allowing us to address and shift these dynamics.

To explore how we can become entangled in the Drama Triangle, let's examine each role more closely and see how they may show up in everyday situations. As you read, consider how these roles may have appeared in your relationships or the relationships of those around you.

1. The Victim: "It's Not My Fault"

The Victim role is characterized by a sense of helplessness and feeling overwhelmed by life's challenges. People in this role often believe they have no control over their circumstances, which can lead them to seek sympathy and support without taking responsibility for changing their situation.

Examples:

- **Personal Relationships:** A person struggling with chronic pain from fibromyalgia may feel defeated by their symptoms, believing there's nothing they can do to alleviate their suffering. They may feel reliant on others to accommodate their needs but resist exploring potential lifestyle or emotional adjustments that might help them manage their condition.

- **Work Environment:** An employee who constantly complains about feeling undervalued or overwhelmed but never takes steps to communicate their needs or seek ways to manage their workload. Instead, they passively accept their situation and look to others for validation, reinforcing their role as a victim of circumstance.

- **Health and Well-Being:** An individual who avoids proactive health steps, like exploring stress management or dietary changes, believing their health issues are solely the result of external factors. They may express frustration but feel powerless to make changes, attributing their condition to factors beyond their control.

The Victim role can lead to chronic stress, resignation, and a sense of defeat. This mindset may manifest physically as fatigue or persistent pain, particularly in conditions like fibromyalgia, where feeling overwhelmed and disempowered can exacerbate symptoms.

2. The Persecutor: "It's Your Fault"

The Persecutor blames others and often acts out of frustration or anger. They may feel justified in their criticisms, believing others are responsible for their unhappiness or challenges. This role can be subtle, such as being overly critical, or more overt, such as lashing out in anger.

Examples:

- **Personal Relationships:** Someone with chronic pain may take out their frustration on a partner, blaming them for not understanding or being supportive enough. They may feel entitled to their anger because they believe their loved ones don't fully appreciate their struggle.
- **Work Environment:** An employee who, when stressed, lashes out at colleagues, blaming them for inefficiencies. They might say, "If others did their job, I wouldn't be so overwhelmed." This attitude alienates coworkers and creates additional tension.
- **Health and Well-Being:** A person who blames doctors, alternative practitioners, or even family members for not providing the "right" solutions. They might say, "No one understands this illness," while resisting exploring changes they could make in their own mindset or lifestyle.

This role is often rooted in a need for control but can lead to additional conflict and isolation. For those dealing with fibromyalgia, the Persecutor role may amplify stress, prevent self-reflection, and hinder the individual's ability to address their own emotional needs.

3. The Rescuer: "Let Me Help You"

On the surface, the Rescuer role may appear helpful, but it can be just as damaging. The Rescuer feels compelled to help others, often to the detriment of their own well-being. While they believe they are being selfless, their help may enable others to stay in their Victim role, preventing real growth.

Examples:

- **Personal Relationships:** A partner who takes on all responsibilities for someone dealing with chronic pain, believing they must "save" them. This can unintentionally reinforce the Victim role, as the individual with fibromyalgia may feel disempowered or dependent, preventing them from exploring self-management strategies.
- **Work Environment:** A coworker who constantly takes on tasks for others, believing they're the only one who can do them properly. While they feel indispensable, they may start resenting others for their perceived lack of competence.
- **Health and Well-Being:** Someone who continually advises others on health and wellness without tending to their own needs. They may say, "You need to take better care of yourself," while neglecting their own health, leading to burnout and resentment.

The Rescuer's behaviour often stems from a desire to feel needed but can lead to exhaustion and frustration. By "rescuing" others, they prevent those individuals from developing self-reliance, while neglecting their own needs.

Breaking Free from the Drama Triangle

Getting caught in the Drama Triangle is exhausting and harmful to both relationships and health. Breaking free requires self-awareness, responsibility, and a commitment to making positive changes.

- **Awareness:** Recognizing your own patterns is the first step. Which role do you gravitate towards, and in what situations? Do you find yourself blaming others, feeling like life is happening to you, or trying to save others even when it's not necessary?
- **Responsibility:** Taking ownership of your role doesn't mean blaming yourself but understanding that you have the power to change your responses.
- **Healthy Alternatives:** Instead of falling into the Victim role, embrace empowerment by acknowledging your feelings and taking proactive steps. Instead of the Persecutor, practice compassionate

communication. Rather than rescuing, offer support only when requested and appropriate, allowing others to take responsibility for their growth.

Escaping the Drama Triangle can feel challenging, but it is essential for healthier relationships and well-being. By identifying and shifting out of these roles, you can foster a profound change in how you interact with others and feel physically and emotionally. Breaking free from these patterns not only supports personal growth but can also ease the emotional burdens that may contribute to chronic health conditions like fibromyalgia.

The Value of Professional Guidance

Breaking old patterns often requires more than awareness—it requires action, support, and sometimes the guidance of a skilled practitioner. Admitting the need for help can be daunting, especially when it triggers insecurities about independence and strength. However, seeking support is a courageous step that can significantly accelerate healing and transformation.

A professional can offer perspective, tools, and techniques that facilitate lasting change. This support is not about dependency but rather about empowering you to understand and resolve deeper conflicts that may be affecting your health. Sometimes, the most profound strength lies not in enduring alone but in reaching out for the support that can help you break free from old patterns and become the healthiest, most empowered version of yourself.

As you move forward on this journey, consider the impact that working with a skilled coach or practitioner could have on your progress. Real growth often involves acknowledging when it's time to seek guidance, allowing you to step confidently into a healthier, more fulfilled life.

Moving from Shadows to Empowerment:

In the earlier part of this book, we explored the stories of Sam, Rachel, Lena, and Clara—four women navigating different emotional conflicts, each expressing aspects of their shadow selves and playing roles within the Drama Triangle. These dynamics, explored through the perspectives of German New Medicine (GNM) and META-Health, reveal how unresolved emotional conflicts can manifest in physical symptoms, including chronic pain and fatigue, often seen in conditions like fibromyalgia.

- **Sam**, embodying the Placator shadow, was quick to put others' needs above her own, often sacrificing her well-being in an effort to please and avoid conflict. This led her to the Rescuer role, constantly trying to manage the needs of her family and colleagues while ignoring her own. Her self-devaluation and fear of disappointing others fuelled her fibromyalgia symptoms, particularly her chronic fatigue and muscle pain.

- **Rachel** lived as the Blamer, frequently projecting responsibility onto others to deflect her own feelings of inadequacy and avoid vulnerability. Often taking on the Persecutor role, she struggled with resentment and control issues, which compounded her emotional stress and contributed to the physical manifestations of chronic pain and tension within her body.

- **Lena**, as the Computer, relied heavily on logic and control, using intellect as a shield from her emotions. Her detachment led her into the Victim role, where she found herself unable to process the emotional shocks of her father's death and a breakup. This unresolved emotional stress triggered cycles of fatigue and pain, as her body reacted to the suppressed conflict.

- **Clara**, embodying the Distractor shadow, used humour and constant activity as a means of avoiding deeper emotions. By filling her life with distractions, she avoided addressing her underlying feelings of inadequacy. She frequently cycled between roles in the Drama Triangle, from Victim to Rescuer to Persecutor, never fully confronting her emotional pain, which intensified her fibromyalgia symptoms.

Each of these women cycled through their shadow behaviors and Drama Triangle roles, unknowingly amplifying emotional and physical conflicts.

However, these shadows and roles can be transformed into empowered versions that promote healing, growth, and emotional stability.

Empowered Versions of the Drama Triangle

- **From Victim to Creator:** Rather than feeling powerless, the Creator takes responsibility and shapes their reality with purpose. Lena could transform her emotional detachment into ownership of her feelings, creating new outcomes by embracing vulnerability and moving toward personal agency.
- **From Persecutor to Challenger:** The Challenger fosters growth through accountability rather than blame. Rachel, instead of blaming others, could challenge herself and those around her to grow without deflecting responsibility, bringing constructive energy into her interactions.
- **From Rescuer to Coach:** The Coach empowers others to find solutions for themselves. Sam, who often sacrificed her needs to care for others, could become a Coach by encouraging others to take responsibility while setting her own boundaries and honouring her needs.

Empowered Versions of the Shadow Selves

- **From Blamer to Warrior:** Rachel's Blamer shadow can evolve into the Warrior, who faces challenges with courage and accountability. Rather than deflecting, the Warrior stands strong, taking action and protecting her values with integrity.
- **From Placator to Lover:** Sam's Placator can shift to the Lover, who values self-care and sets healthy boundaries. The Lover nurtures relationships without sacrificing her identity, finding strength in self-acceptance and balance.
- **From Computer to Guru:** Lena's Computer shadow can grow into the Guru, balancing intellect with emotional insight. The Guru values both reason and feelings, fostering connections that allow for deeper understanding.
- **From Distractor to Jester:** Clara's Distractor can transform into the Jester, who uses humour to face life's difficulties while remaining present with her emotions. The Jester encourages light-heartedness without avoiding underlying truths.

Integrating Empowerment: A Path to Healing

Reflecting on these stories, it's clear that each woman's shadow and Drama Triangle role contributed to her emotional and physical challenges. But by shifting from shadow to empowerment—transforming the Victim into the Creator or the Blamer into the Warrior—there's hope for healing and growth.

For the reader, this journey of transformation is about recognizing the shadow patterns you may see in yourself and understanding that these behaviors don't define you. By embracing the empowered versions of these roles, you can begin to rewrite your story, just as Sam, Rachel, Lena, and Clara could have done.

Reach out for help.

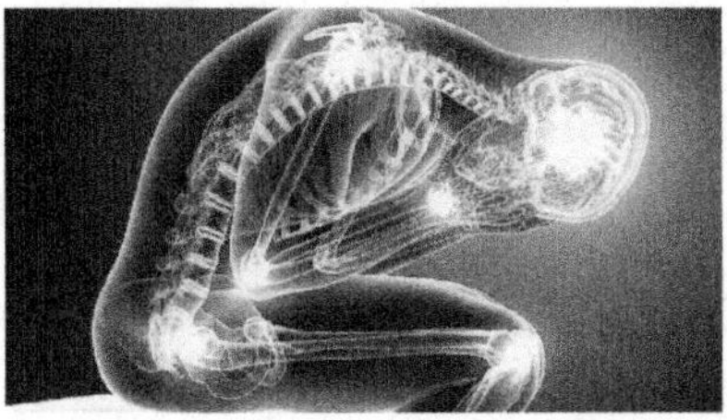

Embracing Support: A Vital Step Towards True Strength

You've come a long way, delving into the complexities of your health, emotions, and overall well-being. Now, as you stand on the threshold of deeper healing, consider a powerful and courageous step: reaching out for support.

Imagine what it would feel like to take full ownership of your health journey, breaking free from old patterns, and moving beyond the limitations that have held you back. You've already begun this transformation by gaining awareness and insight into the root causes of your challenges. Now, ask yourself: Isn't it time to take the next step?

For many, especially those facing chronic conditions like fibromyalgia, the thought of seeking help can feel daunting. It might even feel like an admission of defeat. But what if reaching out wasn't a sign of weakness, but rather a profound expression of your strength? What if asking for support is the very key that unlocks a new level of resilience and inner power?

It's essential to remember that fibromyalgia—or any chronic health issue—is not a random malfunction. Rather, it's your body's way of responding to unresolved emotional conflicts, unspoken needs, and patterns of stress that have been carried for too long. These symptoms, painful as they may be, are your body's attempt to restore balance and bring attention to the areas in your life that need healing. When you address these root issues, when you look at the unprocessed emotions or conflicts beneath them, you open the door to long-lasting health and relief.

You are not powerless. By understanding your emotions and working through unresolved issues, you can regain control over your well-being. These health challenges, though difficult, are part of a meaningful process that can be positively influenced by addressing the emotional and psychological layers involved.

Now, imagine how different things could be with the right support beside you. Picture yourself breaking through barriers and releasing the deeply rooted tensions that have been weighing you down. Imagine the sense of relief and empowerment that comes from having someone who listens, understands, and guides you through your journey with empathy and expertise.

So why not take that next step? What if true strength lies not just in independence, but in the wisdom to know when to seek help? Reaching out is not a surrender—it's an empowered choice, a commitment to invest in yourself and your well-being. When these emotional conflicts are acknowledged and resolved, they create a ripple effect of healing across your life, opening up space for greater peace, energy, and purpose.

In the back of this book, you'll find a list of dedicated coaches and practitioners who are passionate about helping individuals like you. They have the skills, knowledge, and compassion to guide you in reclaiming your health, vitality, and joy. Why not make that investment in yourself? After all, there is no greater investment than the one you make in your own well-being.

If not now, when? If not you, who? It's time to rewrite your story, to step beyond fear and hesitation. Embrace the support available to you, because you deserve it. And remember, true strength lies not in never needing help, but in knowing when to reach out for it.

Summary: Embracing a New Path to Healing and Understanding

Throughout this journey, we've explored fibromyalgia through a transformative lens. Moving beyond conventional perspectives, this book invites you to see chronic pain, fatigue, and other symptoms not as malfunctions but as meaningful responses rooted in emotional conflicts, self-perception, and past experiences. The principles of German New Medicine (GNM) provide a powerful framework, helping us recognize how our mind, emotions, and body are deeply connected in a way that directly impacts our health.

1. **The Foundation of German New Medicine**
   Dr. Ryke Geerd Hamer's revolutionary work has shown that our bodies react to significant emotional shocks through specific biological programs. With the Five Biological Laws as a guide, GNM explains how unresolved conflicts lead to physical manifestations and how addressing these conflicts allows the body to naturally enter a healing phase.

2. **The Role of Shadows and Archetypes**
   We explored the influence of the shadow self—hidden aspects of our personalities like the Blamer, Placator, Computer, and Distractor—and their empowered counterparts. Understanding these shadows reveals how our unmet needs and coping mechanisms can contribute to cycles of stress and chronic symptoms. Embracing empowered roles like the Warrior, Lover, Guru, and Jester allows for personal growth, resilience, and deeper emotional healing.

3. **The Drama Triangle and Empowerment**
   We delved into the Drama Triangle, where roles like Victim, Persecutor, and Rescuer can perpetuate toxic dynamics. By shifting to empowered roles, we break free from these patterns, fostering healthier relationships and inner peace.

4. **Integrating the Six Human Needs**
   Drawing from Tony Robbins' Six Human Needs—certainty, variety, significance, love and connection, growth, and contribution—we looked at how to meet our needs in constructive ways. When balanced, these needs bring stability, resilience, and fulfillment, creating a foundation for lasting health.

5. **A New Understanding of Microbes in Healing**
   The Fourth Biological Law redefines microbes as allies in the healing

process, actively aiding recovery once a conflict is resolved. In fibromyalgia, bacteria, fungi, and viruses assist in tissue repair, emphasizing the body's natural ability to restore balance.

6. **The Quintessence of Healing**
   The Fifth Biological Law, or Quintessence, reinforces that symptoms are not errors but responses with purpose. This law reminds us that our bodies are intrinsically designed for healing when given the chance to address unresolved emotional pain.

As you move forward, remember that fibromyalgia is not an enemy but a signal—a call to explore your inner world and release the conflicts that may be holding you back. Through self-awareness, emotional resilience, and a compassionate understanding of the body-mind connection, healing becomes not just possible but deeply empowering. This is the invitation of German New Medicine: to see your body not as broken but as an intelligent system guiding you toward wholeness.

Recommended Books

"The Human Reboot: Demystifying the Placebo Effect, Spontaneous Remission, and the Emotional Roots of Illness" by Chris Whalley
In The Human Reboot, Chris Whalley delves deep into the emotional roots of illness and the power of the mind in healing. This comprehensive guide connects alternative healing perspectives, such as German New Medicine, META-Health, and Tony Robbins' Six Human Needs, to provide insights into how unresolved emotional conflicts can manifest as physical symptoms. With practical exercises and transformative insights, this book empowers readers to reclaim their health by understanding and addressing the emotional causes of dis-ease. Ideal for those seeking to understand the connection between emotions and physical health, and to embrace a more empowered approach to healing.

"Terminal Cancer Is a Misdiagnosis: Discover a Palliative Care Alternative Medicine You Can Survive" by Danny Carroll
In this thought-provoking book, Danny Carroll explores how conventional medical diagnoses of terminal cancer can be misleading. He provides insights into alternative treatments and perspectives that challenge the traditional view of terminal illness. This book is ideal for anyone seeking hope and exploring alternatives to conventional cancer treatment.

"HAMER: The True Story of Dr. Ryke Geerd Hamer"
This book delves into the life and discoveries of Dr. Ryke Geerd Hamer, the founder of German New Medicine (GNM). It explores his revolutionary ideas about the connection between emotional conflicts and physical disease, challenging conventional medical practices. An essential read for anyone interested in understanding the foundations of GNM and how emotional healing can impact health.

"The Body Keeps the Score: Brain, Mind, and Body in the Healing of Trauma" by Bessel van der Kolk
This book delves into how trauma affects the body and mind and offers methods for healing. It's particularly relevant for women dealing with emotional conflicts tied to health challenges and provides a deep understanding of how trauma manifests physically.

"Radical Remission: Surviving Cancer Against All Odds" by Kelly A. Turner
This book explores the common factors among cancer survivors who have

defied medical odds. Through the stories of patients who experienced radical remissions, Turner highlights essential lifestyle changes and emotional healing practices that have played a role in their recovery.

"Daring Greatly: How the Courage to Be Vulnerable Transforms the Way We Live, Love, Parent, and Lead" by Brené Brown
Brené Brown explores the power of vulnerability and how embracing it can lead to deeper connections and personal growth. This book is relevant for women seeking emotional resilience and strength in the face of health challenges.

"Radical Acceptance: Embracing Your Life With the Heart of a Buddha" by Tara Brach
This book offers practical tools for accepting yourself fully and embracing your life's challenges. It's perfect for women working through emotional conflicts and health issues, teaching how to overcome fear, self-judgment, and shame.

"Goddesses Never Age: The Secret Prescription for Radiance, Vitality, and Well-Being" by Christiane Northrup
This book is a celebration of the wisdom and strength of women as they age. Dr. Northrup provides tips for staying healthy, vibrant, and radiant, physically and emotionally, regardless of age or health challenges.

"You Can Heal Your Life" by Louise Hay
This classic book emphasizes the power of affirmations and positive thinking in healing from physical illness, including cancer. Louise Hay's approach aligns well with the emotional and psychological perspectives in your book.

"The Four Agreements: A Practical Guide to Personal Freedom" by Don Miguel Ruiz
Ruiz outlines four principles for personal freedom: Be impeccable with your word, don't take anything personally, don't make assumptions, and always do your best. It's a powerful book for women seeking to live with integrity and purpose.

"The Drama of the Gifted Child: The Search for the True Self" by Alice Miller
Miller explores how childhood experiences shape our adult lives and how reclaiming the true self can lead to healing and personal transformation.

"Letting Go: The Pathway of Surrender" by David R. Hawkins
Hawkins provides a method for releasing negative emotions and patterns that hold us back. It's a guide for those seeking emotional freedom and spiritual growth.

"The Denial of the True Self" by Alexander Lowen
Lowen discusses the psychological roots of self-denial and how it impacts mental and physical health. This book is for anyone interested in understanding the deeper psychological barriers that prevent them from living authentically.

"The Wisdom of Insecurity: A Message for an Age of Anxiety" by Alan Watts
Watts explores how our pursuit of security leads to suffering and how embracing uncertainty and living in the present can bring peace and fulfillment. It's a profound book for those interested in mindfulness and self-acceptance.

Directory: Trusted Practitioners & Coaches

Dr. Melissa Sell, DC (USA)
Chiropractor, GNM educator/ expert
www.drmelissasell.com

Kora Klapp (Spain)
META-Health Master Practitioner and Trainer
www.metahealth4u.com

Jo Brown (UK)
Coach and Therapy Practitioner
Strategic intervention Coach
Www.BulliedToBulletproof.com

Andi Locke Mears (USA)
ND, MA, CWHE
GNM Practitioner and educator/expert
Www.andilockemears.com

Katherine Willow (Canada)
Mind-Body Medicine including GNM
www.ecowellness.com

Danielle Henderson (USA)
Grief and traumatic events resolution
Strategic Intervention Coach
www.Hope.health.freedom@gmail.com

Avnita Suri (UK)
META-Health Speciality (musculoskeletal pain)
www.avnitasuri.com

Tracy Fance (UK)
Mind Body & Spiritual Coach
www.tracyfance.com

Lishui Springford (Canada)
B.Sc. German New Medicine
Practitioner and teacher
www.mindtreehealth.net

Veronika Kimmich (Australia)
Strategic interventionist and naturopath
www.vmknaturopath.com

Tess Vergara (USA)
Strategic intervention Coach
Soul Realignment
www.tessvergara.com

Jo Stallard (UK)
Strategic Intervention Coach
Hypnotherapy
www.jostallard.co.uk

Desri Goodwin
Strategic Intervention
www.Thetherapyhaven.com

Chris Whalley (UK) Author
Strategic intervention Coach
Meta-Health (GNM) Practitioner, NLP
Timeline
www.decisivecoachinguk.co.uk

Lucia Franziska (Germany)
META-Health Practitioner
Tapping, EFT, NLP, Hypnosis, Yoga, Massage Therapy
www.LuciaFranziska.com

Jo Mason (UK)
META-Health Master Practitioner
EFT, Matrix Reimprinting, PSYCH-K
www.freeyourmindsolutions.com

Elena Dieter-Leibrock (Germany)
META-Health Practitioner
Tapping, Breathing techniques, Mindfulness, Reflexology, herbalist, cosmetics
www.gioiaharmonie.com

Sue Woodriffe
META-Health Practitioner
Tapping, EFT, Matrix Reimprinting, Reiki
www.suewoodriffe.co.uk

Cristina Maggi (Canada)
META-Health Master Practitioner
Tapping, EFT, Reiki, Breathing techniques, re-connection
almaggi71.wixsite.com/cmaggimetahealth

Mohamed Essa (Saudi Arabia)
META-Health Master Practitioner
www.mohamedessa.com

Iris Brennenstuhl (Germany)
META-Health Master Practitioner
www.irisbrennenstuhl.com/

Robert Waghmare (UK)
META-Health Master Practitioner
Tapping, EFT, Matrix Reimprinting, NLP, Hypnosis, Breathing techniques, Mindfulness, Kinesiology, META-Kinetics, Access Consciousness, TBA
www.metahealthacademy.com

Kwesi Anan Odum (UK, Germany)
META-Health Master Trainer
Homeopathy, Colour-Psychology, Categorical Medicine, Astro-Medicine, 64keys, Landmark Communication Model
www.metahealthacademy.com/dr-kwesi/

Dr. Stéphane Provencher (USA)
META-Health Master Practitioner
Physician / medical doctor, Chiropractor, Physician / medical doctor, PhD, PScD, FIM, FICS, BCHHP, BCAMP, CHC, CHLP, CBT
Methods:
Ayurveda, Homeopathy, Tapping, EFT, Reiki, NLP, Hypnosis, Breathing techniques, Kinesiology, SOT Method,Craniopathy
www.ghhcenter.com

Dan Lustig (ISRAEL)
META-Health Master Practitioner & Certification Trainer
EFT, Matrix Reimprinting, NLP
selfheal.co.il/

Craig Weiner (USA)
META-Health Foundation Trainer, META-Health Modality Trainer

Tapping, EFT, Matrix Reimprinting
www.efttappingtraining.com

Lisa Næblerød (Denmark)
META-Health Practitioner
Psychotherapist
simple-being.dk/

John Rhodes (Denmark)
META-Health Master Practitioner
META-Health Trainer
Tapping, NLP, Hypnosis, Kinesiology, BWRT
www.rhodes.nu

Thorsten Krüger
META-Health Practitioner
Homeopathy, NLP
www.barefoot-coaching.com

Susan Gardner (UK)
META-Health Master Practitioner
Tapping, EFT, MET, Reiki, Breathing techniques, Mindfulness
www.metawellbeing.com/

Robyn Harris (UK)
META-Health Practitioner
EFT, Matrix Reimprinting, Reiki, Mindfulness
www.equenergy.com/

Miho Nonami (Japan)
META-Health Master Practitioner
EFT, Reiki, The Journey, META-Kinetics
metamedicinejp.com/

Jasmina Kovacev (NZ)
META-Health Master Practitioner
Tapping, EFT, TAT, NLP, Psycho-oncology, Consciousness Technologies
www.TehnikaEmocionalneSlobode.com

Dr Anu Mehta (India)
META-Health Master Practitioner
PHD in philosophy, Tapping, EFT, Matrix Reimprinting
metahealthindia.co.in

Catherine Koch (Germany)
META-Health Master Practitioner
META-Health Trainer, Tapping, EFT, MET
www.catherine-schmetterling.de/

Caroline Dawson (Australia)
META-Health Practitioner
Tapping, EFT, Matrix Reimprinting, Reiki
www.efttraining.com.au

Ann Bowditch (Guensey)
META-Health Practitioner
Tapping, EFT, Matrix Reimprinting, Hypnosis, Colour Mirrors, Author
www.hypnotherapy.gg/

Aisling Killoran (Ireland)
META-Health Master Practitioner
Tapping, EFT, Matrix Reimprinting, TAT, NLP, Hypnosis, Somatic Experiencing, Breathing techniques, Mindfulness, Hypnosis, HeartMath, EMDR, Fertility Support, Counselling Skills, CBT
www.accomplishchange.com/

Core Models:

German New Medicine

The Learning GNM website is dedicated to bringing the groundbreaking medical discoveries of Dr. med. Ryke Geerd Hamer to the attention of health professionals and the public at large.

www.learninggnm.com/home.html

Meta Health International

www.meta-health.info/

Strategic Intervention

(also known as SI) is a project dedicated to extracting the most practical and effective forms of strategic action and communication from a variety of disciplines: Ericksonian therapy, strategic family therapy, Human Needs Psychology, organizational psychology, neurolinguistics, psychology of influence, strategic studies, traditions of diplomacy and negotiation, and others.

www.rmtcenter.com

The Drame Triangle

www.karpmandramatriangle.com

Jungian Psychology

www.jung.org

Other Useful Resources

YouTube Channels

Mellisa Sell
www.youtube.com/@DrMelissaSell
Here you will find a wealth of amazing videos.

Training

www.andilockemears.com

Andi Locke Mears offers full training in GNM

Thank you for reading! I hope this book has provided you with valuable insights on health, healing, and personal transformation. If you found this book helpful, please consider leaving a review on Amazon. Your feedback helps me to continue improving and reaching more readers just like you.

Stay connected and receive updates on future books, articles, and events by visiting my website at www.decisivecoachinguk.co.uk

or following me on www.facebook.com/decisivemindcoach

Copyright Page

Chris Whalley
www.decisivecoachinguk.co.uk

Want more? Sign up for my newsletter and be the first to hear about new releases, exclusive content, and bonus materials!

Edition
First Edition

Publishing Platform

Published by Kindle Direct Publishing (KDP)

Disclaimer

The information contained in this book is for educational and informational purposes only. It is not intended as medical advice and should not be used as a substitute for professional medical consultation, diagnosis, or treatment. Always seek the advice of your physician or another qualified health provider with any questions you may have regarding a medical condition. The author, Chris Whalley, assumes no responsibility or liability for any damages or negative consequences resulting from the use of any information presented in this book.

All views and opinions expressed in this book are those of the author and do not reflect the views of any organizations or individuals mentioned.

Printed in Great Britain
by Amazon

61185394R00070